Anthropology of the Brain

M000289973

In this unique exploration of the mysteries of the human brain, Roger Bartra shows that consciousness is a phenomenon that occurs not only in the mind but also in an external network, a symbolic system. He argues that the symbolic systems created by humans in art, language, in cooking, or in dress, are the key to understanding human consciousness. Placing culture at the centre of his analysis, Bartra brings together findings from anthropology and cognitive science and offers an original vision of the continuity between the brain and its symbolic environment. The book is essential reading for neurologists, cognitive scientists, and anthropologists alike.

ROGER BARTRA is Professor Emeritus at the University of Mexico (UNAM), and an honorary research fellow at Birkbeck, University of London.

Anthropology of the Brain

Consciousness, Culture, and Free Will

Roger Bartra

Translated by
Gusti Gould

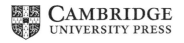
CAMBRIDGE
UNIVERSITY PRESS

CAMBRIDGE
UNIVERSITY PRESS

University Printing House, Cambridge CB2 8BS, United Kingdom

Cambridge University Press is part of the University of Cambridge.

It furthers the University's mission by disseminating knowledge in the pursuit of
education, learning and research at the highest international levels of excellence.

www.cambridge.org
Information on this title: www.cambridge.org/9781107629820

© Roger Bartra 2014

First published 2014

Printed in the United Kingdom by Clays, St Ives plc

A catalogue record for this publication is available from the British Library

ISBN 978-1-107-06036-4 Hardback
ISBN 978-1-107-62982-0 Paperback

Contents

vi   Contents

Preface

In this book I try to explain the mystery of consciousness. Explaining the enigma is not the same thing as *solving* it. I want to tap into, to put forward from the anthropologist's viewpoint, the extraordinary advances in the sciences dedicated to exploring the brain. Neurologists and psychiatrists are convinced that mental processes reside in the brain. My intention is to take an anthropological journey inside the cranium in search of consciousness, or at least of the traces it has left imprinted on the neuronal networks. What can an anthropologist discover in the brain? Identity is one of anthropology's favorite and most studied topics, a condition usually seen as a host of symbols and cultural processes that centers around the definition of an "I," a self that is essentially expressed as an individual fact, but that acquires a variety of collective dimensions: ethnic, social, religious, national, sexual, and many other identities. What identity is there inside the brain? Its principal expression is consciousness.

So that my objective is clear to the reader from the start, I wish to explain my understanding of consciousness – not with a strict definition, but rather by referring to the perspective of a philosopher who, to my way of thinking, is the founder of modern thought on this subject. I am not referring to Descartes. Scientists usually turn to him more to criticize his dualism than to support his ideas: by using him as a reference they remain trapped in the coordinates he established about the relation between the body and the soul. Actually, Descartes used the Latin term *conscientia* very few times. I intend to bring John Locke to my aid. He audaciously used the concept to put forward an idea that provoked intense discussion for a number of decades. I believe his idea is still useful for identifying and circumscribing the problem of consciousness.

When he added a new chapter on consciousness to the second 1694 edition of his *Essay concerning human understanding*, Locke profoundly perturbed the moral and religious traditions of his day.[1] He rejected the orthodox religious view that personal identity is a permanent substance. For Locke the self is not defined by the identity of substances, whether they are divine, material, or infinite: the self is defined by consciousness. Personal identity is based on having consciousness,

---

[1] The book to read about these repercussions is *Locke and the Scriblerians* by Christopher Fox.

something inseparable from thought: "it being impossible for any one to perceive, without perceiving, that he does perceive."[2] Locke does not conceive of consciousness as an immaterial thinking substance and concludes that the soul does not define identity.[3] Less than half a century after the publication of *The passions of the soul* (1649) by Descartes, Locke states that consciousness is the appropriation of things and acts that have to do with the "I" and that are attributable to this self.[4] The self is situated in the identity of a *possession of consciousness*, of a way of behaving.[5] For Locke the word person is a "forensic" term that implies forum: the "I" is responsible, it recognizes acts and attributes them to itself. The soul, in contrast, is indifferent to material surroundings and independent of all matter.[6]

When discussing consciousness, it seems much more stimulating to use Locke as a starting point rather than Descartes. Consciousness can be understood as a series of individual human acts in the context of a social forum that involve a relation between recognition and appropriation of facts and ideas for which the self is responsible. The way in which Locke sees consciousness is closer to the etymological roots of the word: consciousness comes from knowing *with* others. It is socially shared knowledge.[7]

In their desire to place the problem on a level that can be explored scientifically, many neurobiologists have reduced consciousness to a synonym for the fact of noticing, realizing or perceiving the environment. Christof Koch does this in his very useful panoramic summary of the advances in the neurosciences on the study of consciousness. For him *awareness* is the same as *consciousness*.[8] This automatically blocks all research based on a Lockean understanding of consciousness, an understanding that includes the connection of the "I" with its related surroundings. The advantage the neurobiologists see in broadening the concept of consciousness to include every state of awareness that allows an organism to perceive its environment is that it makes it possible to study the phenomenon in non-human animal species and carry out experiments that are inadmissible in people. However, by excluding the cultural networks that envelop the consciousness of the self, even strictly neuronal phenomena become clouded. They are limited to being understood only in that broader sense. I would like to emphasize the fact that throughout the book I will understand consciousness as the process of being conscious of being conscious. A Castilian dictionary from the seventeenth

---

[2] Locke, *An essay concerning human understanding*, chapter 27, § 9.

[3] *Ibid.*, chapter 27, §§ 12 and 15.   [4] *Ibid.*, chapter 27, § 16, pp. 324–325.

[5] *Ibid.*, chapter 27, § 23, p. 328.   [6] *Ibid.*, chapter 27, § 27, p. 332.

[7] The roots of the Latin term *conscius* are *scive* (know) and *con* (with). The Oxford English Dictionary gives: "knowing something with others."

[8] Koch, *The quest for consciousness*, p. 3. With more precision the neurobiologist Francisco Javier Álvarez Leefmans has defined consciousness as "a mental process, in other words, neuronal, through which we notice our "I" and its environment, as well as its reciprocal interactions in the realm of time and space;" "La conciencia desde una perspectiva biológica," p. 17.

century produced the following definition: "Consciousness is the science of the self, or very certain science and quasi-certainty of that which is in our spirit, good or bad."[9] I like the naïve conviction with which this antiquated definition accepts that science can know the secrets of the self, whether benign or malignant, with certainty.

Where do my reflections on the problem of consciousness come from? I can refer to at least four principal sources. First are my many years as a sociologist immersed in the study of different expressions of social consciousness and their relation to the structures that drive it. Second are my anthropological studies of history and the function of myths, emphasizing those that deal with mental illness or identity. Third, I cultivate the habits of introspection, sometimes systematically, but more often randomly following the fluctuations of my literary and musical tastes or my reveries.[10] Finally, and very importantly, I spent a number of years reading and studying the results of research carried out by neuroscientists. I believe I have brought together enough elements to present a tentative and exploratory essay, undoubtedly risky and rash, on one of the greatest enigmas facing science.[11] I must confess I would never have dared embark on this journey if, while I was walking alone through the Gothic quarter in Barcelona in 1999, a sudden thought had not irrevocably pierced my brain. From that autumn day on, I began to obsessively search through neurological research for the knowledge that would convince me to abandon my line of thinking. I admit I was not displeased – though I was surprised – to discover that what I read helped to strengthen the original idea and to further its trans- formation into a manageable hypothesis. I have not been able to resist the temptation of presenting it to readers in the hope that it just might make a contribution toward solving the enigma that is consciousness.

---

[9] Sebastián de Covarrubias, *Tesoro de la lengua castellana o española* (1611).

[10] Javier Álvarez Leefmans explains the importance of introspection in "La conciencia desde una perspectiva biológica." A similar idea is developed by José Luis Díaz in his article "Subjetividad y método." Díaz rightly states: "if consciousness is not an internal, secret, and hidden mental factor, but is in some way imprinted on verbal information, then it is clear that an empirical and technically credible analysis of introspective verbal information would actually be an analysis of the characteristics of consciousness"(p. 164).

[11] In 2003 I presented my hypothesis on the exocerebrum in a conference at the Centro Cultural Conde Duque in Madrid on November 6. I published my conference paper in February 2004 as "La conciencia y el exocerebro." Another advance notice of my ideas appeared as "El exocer- ebro: una hipótesis sobre la conciencia" in 2005.

Part I

Consciousness and symbolic systems

1   The hypothesis

At the beginning of the third millennium the human brain still remains a mysterious organ unwilling to give up its secrets. Scientists have not yet been able to understand the neuronal mechanisms that sustain thought and consciousness. Many of these functions occur in the cerebral cortex, a tissue that resembles the rind of a large fruit, such as a papaya, that has been squeezed and wrinkled upon being inserted into our cranium. I would like to extract this cortex so that, by unfolding its sulci, I could spread it out like a handkerchief over my desk in front of me to examine its texture. If that were possible, a beautiful grey cloth, two or three handspans wide, would now be lying before my eyes. I could run my gaze over the thin surface, looking for signs that would allow me to decipher the mystery hidden in the network connecting billions of neurons.

Neurobiologists have managed to do something similar. Thanks to the refinement of new methods for observing the nervous system (such as positron emission tomography and functional magnetic resonance imaging) scientists have rapidly advanced their studies of brain functions. In their euphoria they baptized the last ten years of the twentieth century as the "decade of the brain," and many believed they were very close to the solution of one of the greatest mysteries facing science. However, even though colorful images of the marvelous interior landscape of the brain unfolded before our eyes, they were not able to explain the neuronal mechanisms of thought and consciousness.

In one way, scientists approached the problem of human consciousness much like the naturalists of the eighteenth century who were looking for "man in his natural state" in order to understand the naked essence of the human being, stripped of all artificiality hiding it. Is culture responsible for the violence and corruption that dominate humans? Or is there some congenital evil imprinted in the nature of humans themselves? To unravel the mystery of human consciousness, neurology has also attempted to look for the natural biological keys to the functioning of the central nervous system. An effort has been made to rid the brain of the artificial and subjective veils that envelop it in an attempt to answer this question: are consciousness, language, and intelligence the result of culture or are they genetically printed in neuronal circuits?

It has long been known that "man in his natural state" existed only in the imagination of philosophers and naturalists influenced by the Enlightenment. And it can also be suspected that the "naked neuronal man" does not exist either: a human brain in a natural state is fiction. It is understandable and very positive that from the start, the decade of the brain was marked by a strong rejection of Cartesian dualism. Gerald Edelman, one of today's most intelligent neuroscientists, opens his book on the subject of the mind with a critique of Descartes's idea of a thinking substance (*res cogitans*) separated from the body.[1] But the matter became blurred when the rejection of metaphysical thinking substances was converted into a blind disregard for cultural and social processes that most certainly are extracorporeal.

With this in mind, at the end of the decade of the brain, I read Stevan Harnad's intelligent assessment of the attempts to reveal the mystery of consciousness and complex mental functions.[2] This work shows how the decade of the brain made great strides in explaining some aspects of neuronal functioning, but left the problem of consciousness in the dark. This assessment had a powerful effect on me and made me realize that neurobiology had ignored fundamental aspects without which it would be difficult to advance the understanding of that aspect of the mind. I had spent a good part of the decade of the brain studying, as an anthropologist, the medical sciences that had tried to understand the functioning of the human brain during the Renaissance and the dawn of modernity.[3] I was so absorbed in this work that at times I felt as if I were a practicing physician in Salamanca or Paris in the seventeenth century. The doctors of that epoch firmly believed in the Hippocratic and Galenic humoral theories and therefore easily passed from the corporeal microcosmos to the astronomical macrocosmos, agilely traversing the worlds of geography, customs, seasons, food and diet, and the ages. With this background I approached modern-day neurobiology: what would an anthropologist who had returned from a long journey through the Spanish Golden Age be able to understand?

My first impression was the following: neurobiologists are desperately looking for something – consciousness – in the functional structure of the human brain, when it might be found somewhere else.[4] I wish to reiterate that I use the term consciousness when I refer to the consciousness of the self or the consciousness of being conscious. I imagined how a Renaissance doctor, when on this same search, would think that the feeling of being a unique separate particle could be due to

---

[1] Edelman, *Bright air, brilliant fire*. Two years later, Antonio Damasio popularized the critique in his book *Descartes' error*. An example of this dualist interpretation, though somewhat contradictory, can be read in Arturo Rosenblueth's book *Mind and brain*.
[2] Harnad, "No easy way out."   [3] Bartra, *Melancholy and culture*.
[4] In no way do I support Skinner's old complaint in *About behaviourism* that to study the brain was a way to erroneously search for the causes of conduct within the organism, instead of doing so in the outside world.

anxiety produced by a defective function of the pneumatic impulses in the cerebral ventricles, consequently making it impossible to comprehend man's place in Creation. Consciousness would not only be situated in the functioning of the brain but also (and perhaps mainly) in the suffering of a dysfunction.

A motor or pneumatic machine (such as the brain driven by *pneuma* in Galenic medical terminology) is said to "suffer" when it takes on a task that demands more strength than it has and, as a result, stops. As a mental experiment, let us imagine that this pneumatic motor is a "brain in a natural state" dealing with a problem that is beyond its capacity to resolve. This pneumatic motor is subjected to "suffering."

Now, let us suppose that this pneumatic brain abandons its natural state, and it does not turn off or stop, as would happen with a motor limited to using only its "natural" resources. Instead of stopping and remaining stationary in its natural condition, this hypothetical neuronal motor creates a mental prosthesis in order to survive despite intense suffering. This prosthesis does not have a somatic makeup but substitutes weakened somatic functions. It must be immediately pointed out that it is necessary to repress the Cartesian impulses of the seventeenth-century physician: these extrasomatic prostheses are not thinking substances that are separate from the body nor are they supernatural and metaphysical energies or computer programs that can be separated from the body like the Cheshire Cat's smile. The prosthesis is actually a cultural and social network of extrasomatic mechanisms closely connected to the brain. Of course, this search must try to find certain specific cerebral mechanisms that can be connected to the extracorporeal elements.

Let us return to our mental experiment. We must try to explain why a human being (or protohuman), when facing an important challenge – such as a change of habitat – and therefore experiencing acute suffering, creates a powerful individual consciousness instead of becoming paralyzed or dying. Such an event would not occur in the case of a motor (or a fly). The origin of this consciousness is a cultural prosthesis (mainly speech and the use of symbols) that, associated with the use of tools, allows survival in a world that has become excessively hostile and difficult. The circuits of anguished emotions created by the difficulty to survive pass through the extrasomatic spaces of the cultural prostheses, but the neuronal circuits that they connect to become aware of the "outerness" or "strangeness" of those symbolic and linguistic channels. It should be underlined that, seen from this perspective, consciousness is not the becoming aware of the existence of an exterior world (a habitat), but rather is the fact that a portion of that external environment "functions" as if it were part of the neuronal circuits. To put it differently: incapacity and dysfunction in the cerebral somatic circuit are compensated for by cultural functionalities and capacities. That the neuronal circuit is sensitive to the fact it is incomplete and needs an external supplement is its mystery. This sensitivity is part of consciousness.

Antonio Damasio, one of the best researchers described by Harnad, insists on the division between the interior environment, precursor of the individual self, and its external surroundings.[5] It is possible that this belief, deeply rooted among neurobiologists, is an obstacle to advancing the understanding of the physiological fundamental principles of human consciousness. Let us consider a different idea: consciousness would arise from the cerebral capacity to recognize the continuation of an *internal* process in external circuits located in the environment. It is as if a part of the digestive and circulatory mechanism were to artificially occur outside of us. We could contemplate our laminated intestines and veins hooked up to a portable prosthetic apparatus driven by programmed cybernetic systems.

This happens in science-fiction cyborgs and in experiments carried out on primates that, thanks to an implanted electrode, have been able to mentally control a brain-machine connection to move a robotic arm from a distance.[6] On the other hand, we are accustomed to being surrounded by prostheses that help us memorize, calculate, and even encode our emotions. In relation to this, another book appearing at the close of the decade of the brain, written by the philosopher Colin McGinn, uses a very important image that unfortunately was not fully taken advantage of. In his argument for demonstrating that the human brain is incapable of finding a solution to the problem of consciousness, McGinn imagines an organism whose brain, instead of being hidden inside the cranium, is distributed outside its body like a skin. It is an exocerebrum, similar to the exoskeleton of insects and crustaceans.[7] When this organism experiences the color red, its thinking skin, even though exposed to the exterior, is not more easily understood. The "private" character of consciousness, says McGinn, has nothing to do with the fact that our brain is hidden: experiencing the color red is always buried inside a completely inaccessible innerness. McGinn's error lies precisely in believing that consciousness is buried in the interior. If we imagine that the strange creature with a neuronal epidermis is capable of coloring its belly when it thinks about red, and other organisms of the same species can contemplate and identify that, then we are getting closer to our reality: the cultural exocerebrum that we possess really does turn red when we express our experiences with inks and paints of that color. The idea of an external brain was originally outlined by Santiago Ramón y Cajal who, when he proved the extraordinary and precise selectivity of the neuronal networks of the retina, considered them to be a peripheral brain segment.[8]

[5] Damasio, *The feeling of what happens. Body and emotion in the making of consciousness*, pp. 135ff.
[6] Carmena *et al.*, "Learning to control a brain-machine interface for reaching and grasping by primates."
[7] McGinn, *The mysterious flame*, p.11.
[8] In Ramón y Cajal's work "La rétine des vertébrés" he considers the retina to be "a true nervous center, a kind of peripheral brain segment" (p. 121). Today a "second brain" is also spoken of in

I want to go back to the image of the exocerebrum so I can allude to systemic extrasomatic circuits. Different brain systems have been spoken of: the reptilian system, the limbic system, and the neocortex.[9] I believe a fourth level can be added: the exocerebrum. To explain and complement this idea I would like to draw a parallel here inspired by biomedical engineering that builds sensory substitution systems for the blind, the deaf, and for those with other special needs.[10] Thanks to neuronal plasticity, the brain is able to adapt and build circuits, substituting those that function with deficiencies, in areas that are not affected. If we transfer this focus to the exocerebrum we can assume that, in certain hominids, important deficiencies or inadequacies of the coding and classification system arising from an environmental change or from mutations and seriously affecting certain senses (smell, hearing), facilitated their substitution by other areas of the brain closely tied to cultural systems of symbolic and linguistic coding (Broca's and Wernicke's areas). The new condition presents a problem: substitutive neuronal activity cannot be understood without the corresponding cultural prosthesis. This prosthesis can be defined as a symbolic substitution system that would have its origin in a set of compensatory mechanisms that replace those brain functions that have deteriorated or become deficient in the presence of a very different environment. The brain functions are replaced through operations that are based on symbols taken from that external environment. My hypothesis postulates that certain regions of the human brain genetically acquire a neurophysiological dependency on the symbolic substitution system. This system is obviously transmitted by cultural and social mechanisms. It is as if the brain needed the energy of outside circuits in order to synthesize and break down symbolic and imaginary substances in a particular anabolic and catabolic process.

I have used a variety of metaphors for the purpose of simply and briefly explaining a hypothesis on consciousness and the exocerebrum. Now the main idea needs to be separated into its constituent parts so that a careful search for the scientific data to support my interpretation can be undertaken. However, I wanted to express some core ideas in advance so that when we delve into the details we do not lose sight of the original objective.

reference to the enteric nervous system, a network of almost autonomous circuits regulating all facets of digestion from start to finish between the esophagus and colon, including the stomach and all the intestines (Gershon, *The second brain*).

[9] I am referring to the ideas of Paul D. MacLean in *A triune concept of brain and behaviour*. He refers to three types of brain: reptilian, paleomammalian and neomammalian.

[10] Bach-y-Rita, *Brain mechanisms in sensory substitution*.

2   Evolution of the brain

The encephalic mass spread out on my desk as the imaginary handkerchief that could reveal the secrets of the mind takes up a space, when squeezed together, of between 1200 and 1500 cubic centimeters inside the cranium of anatomically modern humans. *Homo erectus*, the ancestor of *Homo sapiens*, who appeared approximately one and a half million years ago, had an encephalic mass whose volume was between 850 and 1100 cubic centimeters. And a much longer time before that, the brain of *Homo habilis*, who appeared about two and a half million years ago, had a volume of between only 510 and 750 cubic centimeters. This evolutionary process began some six million years ago, when a group of large apes evolved, giving rise to different species of bipeds, the australopithecines. For some scientists this period of six million years is too short in evolutionary terms to have resulted in the emergence of the intellectual and cognitive capacities characteristic of *Homo sapiens*. It has been argued that the only mechanism that can explain the rapid evolutionary process is one that is cultural and social in nature. Michael Tomasello maintains that not enough time has passed for there to have been a normal evolutionary process in which genetic variation and natural selection have created, one by one, the cognitive abilities capable of inventing and developing complex technologies and tools, sophisticated forms of representation and symbolic communication, and elaborate social structures that crystallize into cultural institutions.[1]

Even though I am convinced of the huge importance of cultural circuits in the formation of individual consciousness, they should not be seen as the magical solution to the mysteries of the origin of the anatomically modern brain. Tomasello rejects the idea that language was created from a mutation. For him the key lies in the idea that a new intentional manner of identifying with and understanding one another among members of the same species evolved biologically.[2] The continuation of the process, from this unique cognitive adaptation that establishes recognition of others as intentional beings, would have had a completely cultural character and produced the development of symbolic forms of

---

[1] Tomasello, *The cultural origins of human cognition*, pp. 2–4.   [2] *Ibid.*, p. 204.

communication. This development, Tomasello maintains, takes place at a speed unequaled by any process of biological evolution. In contrast, Stephen Jay Gould has stated that there is a sufficient amount of time for a change at the biological level to have occurred. Gould begins by warning against the dangerous trap that defining evolution as a continuous flow implies and states that change takes place by means of the punctuational speciation of isolated subgroups and not through anagenetic change of the entire group at a slow geological rhythm.[3] Gould exposes the mistake of thinking that the growth of cranial capacity that occurred during the period separating *Homo erectus* from *Homo sapiens* represents an example of extraordinary evolutionary velocity, something so rare that it would only be explained by the marvelous adaptation and feedback capacities of human consciousness – or in other words, that the speed of this change would only be explained by the intervention of cultural processes. Actually, the rhythm of change is not extraordinary, but rather it is perfectly normal that the encephalic mass has doubled its size in 100 thousand years (three thousand generations).[4] Gould explains that the change from *Homo erectus* to *Homo sapiens* was a seemingly rapid process of species emergence that probably took place in Africa between 100 and 250 thousand years ago.[5]

We should not focus only on the growth (absolute and relative) of cranial capacity. A study has pointed out the importance of also observing the form the brain adopts, and has discovered the existence of two tendencies in the evolution of the form of the brain in the genus *Homo*. The two processes arrive at a similar size of cranial capacity, in one case the Neanderthal human and in the other the modern human. The first developmental pattern of cranial configuration shows that as size increases, intraparietal distance decreases. This pattern is seen in the evolution from the most archaic specimens up to the Neanderthals. But the process of change resulting in the modern human cranium displays an evolutionary leap that separates it from the pattern just described and marks the beginning of a new trajectory. The new tendency, with the increase in cranial capacity, produces a major parietal expansion resulting in a more spherical configuration (brachycephalic) of the brain. This seems to indicate that the cognitive capacities of the modern human are not a mere expansion of archaic abilities, but rather acquisitions of new aptitudes. Neanderthals and modern humans represent two different and independent evolutionary trajectories.[6]

Into this context it is possible to introduce the hypothesis on how consciousness functions. A relatively isolated and geographically located subgroup of hominids in Africa a quarter of a million years ago experienced rapid changes in the structure, configuration, and size of their central nervous system. These

---

[3] Gould, *The structure of evolutionary theory*, p. 913.   [4] *Ibid.*, pp. 851ff. and 915.
[5] *Ibid.*, p. 916.
[6] Bruner, Manzi, and Arsuaga, "Encephalization and allometric trajectories in the genus *Homo*."

changes were added to transformations, surely many years before, in the vocal apparatus enabling the articulation of speech as we know it today. We can assume that mutations in these archaic hominids affected the functions, form, and size of the cerebral cortex, but also caused transformations in the sensory systems that made it difficult for them to adapt to the environment – perhaps changes in olfactory receptivity and modifications in the ability to localize sound sources, or alterations of olfactory and auditory memories. Their neuronal circuits would be insufficient, and the stereotyped reactions to the accustomed challenges would cease to function well. Perhaps we could also add the fact that important climatic changes and forced migrations exposed them to growing difficulties, putting them at a disadvantage with other hominids that were better adapted to the environment and could respond more quickly to everyday challenges.

The primitive *Homo sapiens* stops recognizing a portion of the signals originating in its surroundings. In the presence of a strange environment, this human suffers, has trouble recognizing roads, objects, or places. To survive it uses new resources found in its brain: it has to mark or signal objects, spaces, crossroads, and the rudimentary instruments it uses. These marks or signals are voices, colors, or figures, true artificial supplements or semantic prostheses that enable it to complete the mental tasks that are causing it such difficulty. In this way it gradually creates an external substitution system of symbols for the atrophied or missing brain circuits, taking advantage of the new capacities acquired during the encephalization and brachycephalic process that has separated early modern humans from their Neanderthal counterparts. An exocerebrum emerges that guarantees a great capacity for adaptation. In other words, the exocerebrum substitutes the disorder caused by confronting a diversity of ecological niches with an order created by a stable symbolic niche.

This interpretation runs into a problem: in the evolutionary process there is a blurred lapse of time separating the emergence of anatomically modern humans and the moment for which we have archaeological records of cultural activity based on learned symbolic communication forms. Adam Kuper has observed that clearly modern humans appeared at least some 60 thousand years before the presence of a developed culture. He therefore assumes that culture came on the scene late, but once it did, cultural evolution advanced at a much faster pace than that dictated by the slow mutations of biological evolution.[7] These changes occurred during the transition from the Middle to the Upper Paleolithic, when the Mousterian lithic industries of the Neanderthals, probably incapable of

---

[7] Kuper, *The chosen primate*, chapter 4. It must be said that evolution is not only a result of gene mutations; molecular biologists agree that biological evolution also includes post-translational modifications, polymorphisms, and the so-called junk DNA. I will not go into these other technical dimensions, but only mention the subject of genetic mutations.

symbolic thought, were substituted by the Aurignacian lithics of the modern Cro-Magnons, humans who possessed language, formed social groups, practiced rituals, and had an organized hunting and gathering economy.

This gap between the acquisition of modern physical features and the development of a symbolic culture can be explained. Ian Tattersall finds the key in the so-called exaptation.[8] Unlike adaptation, it deals with spontaneous innovations that originally had no function or performed a very different role from the one they ended up having. A well-known example is that of feathers, which long before they became useful for flight, served as a layer for maintaining body heat. Tattersall believes that peripheral speech mechanisms were not an adaptation but rather a mutation that occurred several hundred thousand years before they became limited to the function of articulating sounds. And possibly, according to this scientist, the cognitive capacities we possess were also a transformation occurring 100 or 150 thousand years ago that were not taken advantage of (exapted) until 60 or 70 thousand years ago when, in certain archaic humans, a cultural innovation took place that activated the potential to carry out symbolic cognitive processes that had resided in the brain without being used.[9] According to Tattersall, the impetus for this cultural process was the invention of language. Here, he introduces a doubtful hypothesis: he speculates that there was already a neuronal wiring for linguistic ability inscribed in the brain, and the only thing missing for it to start working was the outside stimulus. The trigger could have been as simple as something improvised by a group of children at play. Once this marvelous invention appeared, it would be adopted by the entire society and then passed on to other groups.[10]

Why humans took several tens of thousands of years to discover the potentialities dormant in their brain is not clear. Was it a product of mere chance? That does not seem to be an adequate explanation. I believe we must recognize that neuronal transformation began to have consequences from the moment a subgroup of hominids had to face challenges that demanded resources different from the ones they normally used. The ability to give objects a name was not the random result of a children's game. The important aspect in an exaptation process are the refunctionalizations of non-adaptive modifications that Gould calls spandrels, a term he took from architecture: those unplanned triangular spaces that serve no specific purpose and are the consequence of inserting an arch in a square or the triangular spaces that are formed under a dome when it stands on a set of rounded arches. Cerebral spandrels might have been neuronal circuits open to non-existent functions, useless memories, or external signals that never arrive, or to mechanisms unrelated to cognitive processes. Gould

[8] Tattersall, *The monkey in the mirror*, pp. 51ff. See the first formulation of the concept in Gould and Vrba, "Exaptation – a missing term in the science of form."
[9] Tattersall, *The monkey in the mirror*, pp. 153 and 182.   [10] *Ibid.*, pp. 160–163.

explains that the number of potential spandrels increases considerably in relation to an organism's complexity: their number is limited in the cylindrical umbilical space of the gastropod when compared with the large number stored in the human brain – a considerably higher number of spandrels than the number of adaptive changes occurring as a result of encephalic mass expansion.[11]

My hypothesis on the exocerebrum, as I have stated before, involves a situation in which the individual is subjected to suffering when confronting the difficulties of survival under hostile conditions. I would like to support my argument with the ideas of Antonio Damasio about what could have triggered the development of complex forms of social behavior. In my opinion, he correctly supposes that social and cultural strategies evolved as a way of dealing with suffering in individuals endowed with remarkable capacities to remember and anticipate. The key to Damasio's interpretation lies in the fact that this suffering is something more than the pain an individual feels in the form of a somatosensory signal provoked by a wound, a blow, or a burn. An emotional state that is experienced as suffering follows the pain. Damasio explains that pain is a lever for the adequate deployment of emotional impulses and instincts. Likewise, the organism deploys emotional devices to provide ways of avoiding or easing suffering. Something similar happens in relation to pleasure, a sensation creating additional emotional states.[12]

A further step must be taken: to look for the possible neuronal consequences of suffering under conditions in which the individual does not find the organic means to avoid it. After all, suffering is the result of a deficiency, an absence, a privation. Under these conditions the organism feels the need to replace the resources it lacks: not only does it add an adequate emotional state, but it also resorts to symbolic and cognitive mechanisms that reside in the brain as spandrels lodged above the arches of its neuronal architecture. Of course this can involve the use of weapons and tools, but especially the allocation of words to objects, to emotions or to people, the implementation of signs along the roads or at the source of supplies, the performance of rhythms and ritual movements to symbolize identity and the cohesion of family or tribal groups, and the use of classification techniques as artificial memories.

It is not certain that there has been a void of some 60 thousand years, a strange transition interval during which now anatomically modern humans, endowed with a brain like ours, would have lived without developing the symbolic capacities of beings that more than 30 thousand years ago created the carved ivory figures found in the Hohle Fels cave in the Swabian Alb and the Chauvet cave paintings in the south of France. It is very possible that it is largely an information void that future discoveries may be able to fill. In fact, traces of

---

[11] Gould, *The structure of evolutionary theory*, p. 87.
[12] Damasio, *Descartes' error*, "Post scriptum."

these new discoveries have been found in the Blombos cave excavations in South Africa, where there are possible indications of human symbolic activity from 75 thousand years ago.[13] On the other hand, surely part of the early traces of the most rudimentary cognitive activity made from perishable materials has not survived. The oldest remains of modern human beings associated with the Middle Paleolithic have been found in the south of Africa. The most accepted theory is that *Homo sapiens* originated on that continent and probably arrived in Europe more than 45 thousand years ago when the last glacial period was reaching its lowest temperatures. The human exocerebrum, a set of cultural processes closely connected to the central nervous system, most likely expanded during this period. From these and other indications, Tomasello has said that "the inevitable conclusion is that individual human beings possess a biologically inherited capacity to live culturally."[14] I believe it is more likely that they suffer from a genetically inherited incapacity to live as other animals do – naturally, biologically. This takes us on the search for those neuronal circuits that are characterized by their incomplete nature and that require an extrasomatic supplement.

[13] Henshilwood *et al.*, "Emergence of modern human behavior." Also see Wong, "The morning of the modern mind."
[14] Tomasello, *The cultural origins of human cognition*, p. 53.

3   Brain plasticity

Before beginning to look for incomplete neuronal circuits that require external prostheses in order to function, it is necessary to tackle a broader problem: the form in which cerebral networks are configured to adapt to experiences the individual confronts when interacting with the environment throughout his or her life. Researchers have demonstrated the existence of neuronal plasticity processes in circuits that require experiences coming from the external environment in order to be normally completed in the brains of mammals and other animals. But not all plasticity depends on external factors. It is not simply reduced to the way in which certain cerebral circuits are shaped by the environment. Donald Hebb's classic study published in 1949 shows that neuronal activity itself can strengthen certain synaptic connections when there is simultaneous activity in the presynaptic terminal and in the postsynaptic element of the neuron.[1] A much-cited example of plasticity in Hebbian synapses are the ganglion cells in the mammalian retina that organize layers of the lateral geniculate body in the thalamus of the brain by firing sequences of impulses through the eye. Activity after-effects appear to be randomly produced in both rhythm and direction in such a way that the possibility of cells far away from each other firing simultaneously is remote, and so the connection holding them together becomes weak or disappears. This type of after-effect can still be observed in retinas that are separated from the eye and maintained alive in liquid solutions, which illustrates the independence of these plasticity processes with regard to external stimuli. This type of plasticity enables the genomic flow of information to be reduced, thus explaining how it is possible that the emergence of each neuron and each connection throughout an individual's growth and development would not need to be previously encoded in the genome.[2]

---

[1] Hebb, *The organization of behavior.* A very similar idea was expressed by F. A. Hayek in 1952 in his stimulating book *The sensory order*, a treatise unjustly forgotten that expounds a theory that today should make many neurobiologists reflect, and anticipates ideas that were presented much later by philosophers dedicated to the cognitive sciences.
[2] Schatz, "The developing brain."

Brain plasticity is related to the processes of origin and development of circuits that are not directly determined genetically. Practically all the cells of our organism contain the same genes. Each gene, made of DNA, produces a type of protein that is the substance that our body is basically made up of. But in each kind of cell some genes are turned on and others are turned off: this is why, as has been known for some time, the gene that produces insulin only does so in the pancreas and not in the brain. A more recent discovery is the fact that there are genes that are not permanently turned off or turned on, but rather are activated or deactivated according to experience. This is the case of certain genes in the neurons that do not spend all day doing the same thing. For that reason, proteins in the brain change according to experience.

This leads us to the forms of plasticity in neuronal circuits that require experiences coming from the external environment in order to be completed in a normal fashion. One of the most cited examples is that of the formation of columns corresponding to ocular dominance in the visual cortex. If vision is impeded in one of the eyes in growth-sensitive periods, the corresponding columns do not develop well and they shrink.[3] Studies on the effect of monocular suturing of the eyelid in monkeys and cats have attempted to determine the beginning and end of the period of growth during which the development of columns in the visual cortex is sensitive to external stimuli. The onset itself of the sensitive period appears to be affected by visual impulses. The beginning of the process of ocular dominance formation was delayed in cats that were not allowed to receive visual stimuli in both eyes.[4] In children it is known that cataracts can cause permanent blindness if left untreated, while in human adults they cause only inconvenience until they are removed.[5] Another experiment attempted to demonstrate the influence of movement on visual concept configuration. Two groups of kittens were selected: the first group could move around freely, but dragging a little car carrying a kitten from the second group that was not allowed to move, but had ample vision of the environment. After a time, when all the kittens were freed, the ones that had been moving, pulling the car, behaved normally. But the kittens that had remained immobilized in the car behaved as though they were blind. They bumped into objects and fell off edges. Experience appears to be necessary so that "maps" can be formed in the parietal lobes that enable individuals to be conscious of their surrounding space. The same problem, seen from a different perspective, is revealing: people that have suffered injuries to the parietal lobes are unable to perceive the things that are in a certain area of their visual field (generally the left side). Nevertheless, it has

---

[3] Hubel and Wiesel, "The period of susceptibility to the physiological effects of unilateral eye closure in kittens."

[4] Neville and Bavelier, "Specificity and plasticity in neurocognitive development in humans."

[5] Clifford, "Neural plasticity."

been demonstrated that the objects in the invisible area activate visual cortex neurons while the visible objects also activate certain areas of the prefrontal cortex and the parietal lobes.[6]

The fact that plasticity that is dependent on experience in order to be completed can be combined with other forms of plasticity needs to be underlined. Different studies have shown that spontaneous neuronal activity provides guidelines for constructing circuits in the visual cortex. Experiments carried out on ferrets whose optic nerves were cut without affecting the thalamocortical connection showed that after some seven hours, high frequency thalamic impulses returned in even greater correlated form than normal. This may indicate that the construction of ocular dominance columns does not totally depend on activity generated in the retina.[7]

The examples I have given refer to a type of plasticity that waits for the experience of external stimuli in order to begin. Another form of plasticity must be mentioned that takes us closer to my hypothesis: these are plasticity processes that, even though they do not require outside stimuli, are modified by experience. This form of plasticity refers to neuronal changes that occur as a consequence of learning. William Greenough's experiments have examined this type of plasticity. This researcher and his colleagues raised two separate groups of rats from an early age, from twenty-eight to thirty-two days, in very different environments. The rats from the first group were placed in individual cages and were given only food and water. The second group was put in spacious cages together with other rats; there they had different toys and a wide variety of interesting and changing stimuli that they could freely explore. When their brains were examined one month later, big differences were found: the rats that had been raised in a stimulating environment had 60 percent more multicephalic dendritic spines in the neurons of the striate body.[8] It is possible that multicephalic spines indicate the presence of parallel connections between neurons that could reinforce, weaken, or create connections to new synapses, altering the neuronal map.

There is a particularly revealing example of the changes provoked by the social environment in the brain. A community of cichlid fish called *Haplochromis burtoni* lives in Lake Tanganyika. In their natural habitat two types of males are observed: those that dominate a territory and those that have no territory. Approximately only one out of ten males has a dominant behavior and is distinguished by its brilliant blue or yellow color with a distinctive black stripe over the eye, black vertical bars, a black spot at the tip of the gill cover, and

[6] Vuilleumier *et al.*, "Neural fate of seen and unseen faces in visuospatial neglect: A combined event-related MRI and event-related potential study."
[7] Katz *et al.*, "Activity and the development of the visual cortex: New perspectives."
[8] Clifford, "Neural plasticity."

another large red spot behind it. This spectacular appearance contrasts with the unremarkable and subdued colors that the non-territorial males camouflage themselves with. These males look very much like the females and easily blend into their surroundings. The colorful dominant males aggressively defend their respective territories around food sources; they fight with males of neighboring territories, chase the non-dominant males, and attract the females. The non-dominant males survive by imitating the behavior of the females and blending in with them, although they are frequently discovered and expelled. But there is another peculiarity that distinguishes the dominant males: the neurons in the preoptic area of the ventral hypothalamus that contain gonadotropin-releasing hormone (GnRH) are much larger than those in the females and the non-dominant males. However, this situation is not stable. In the experiments, when a dominant adult male was moved to a community where the other males were bigger, in just four weeks the dominant male became dominated and its GnRH neurons became smaller. Much less time is needed (one week) for GnRH neurons to become larger in a non-dominant male that is placed in a new environment where the other males are smaller. It should be added that not everything is advantageous for the eye-catching active male that dominates a territory: its colors easily attract the attention of predatory birds in such a way that its territorial reign is usually relatively brief. Obviously, social interactions and hierarchy powerfully influence neuronal size.

What is it that determines this extraordinary brain plasticity? Research has indicated the probable existence of a hormone, cortisol, as the mediating signal between the tension animals undergo when their social surroundings change and the physiological processes that increase or decrease neuronal size. Therefore, we would have a circuit or a chain that would include social position, the production of a hormone, its function as a signal for triggering changes in genetic expression and in the configuration of certain types of neurons. The most revealing aspect of this process is that it incorporates endogenous cellular and molecular signals together with exogenous changes into the social relations of dominance in the same circuit.[9] Other studies in animals and in humans have shown the sensitivity and vulnerability of the hippocampus when confronting psychosocial tensions and revealed its plasticity as a response to hormonal changes. A continuous tension caused by a difficult social environment can cause neurogenetic processes in the dentate gyrus to be suppressed and the hippocampal pyramidal neurons to be atrophied.[10]

Now I would like to examine a type of neuronal circuit in which an exogenous feedback process also intervenes. Once the learning period is over, the song of many songbirds manifests a repetitive acoustic structure whose great

[9] Fernald and White, "Social control of brains: From behavior to genes."
[10] McEwen, "Stress, sex, and the structural and functional plasticity of the hippocampus."

stability has nothing to do with the fact that the animal listens to other birds. However, in the case of zebra finches it has been shown that feedback that entails listening to other birds is required, in order for the acoustic structure of their song to remain stable. When deafness was provoked in adult finches it was discovered that their song slowly began to deteriorate. This happens because there is a neuronal feedback circuit. In addition, studies have demonstrated that in these birds there is a circuit in the anterior forebrain that is essential during learning and that modulates neuronal plasticity. This circuit does not form part of the basic motor connections that join the song nucleus (HVc) with the premotor nucleus (RA) that in turn is bound to the areas of vocal control, respiratory neurons, and neurons of the vocal organ musculature. The activity of the forebrain circuit continues after the learning period, is activated during song, and is very sensitive to the social context in which the finches interact. It is a type of mediating circuit between the external environment and the internal plasticity.[11]

The majority of studies on brain plasticity linked to environmental and social surroundings have been directed toward the search for paths that follow the influence of the external environment on the process of modifying neuronal networks. In other words, research has principally observed the process in only one direction: from the outside toward the inside. A stimulating essay by Stephen Kennepohl asks whether a cultural neuropsychology that studies the association between variations in the cultural context and differences in the nervous system, is possible. Cultural factors contribute to shaping the brain in different ways: each culture's own ecological environment could activate certain neuronal connections, childhood learning differentially alters brain development, and adaptation of the brain to new experiences is maintained, although with less flexibility, in the adult.[12] The model is essentially unidirectional, centered on capturing what is outside to deposit its representation (or something similar) into the interior of the brain, thereby provoking modifications in the neuronal connections. The possibility that the channels in the brain through which the influence of culture is conducted could be two-way, forming authentic circuits, is barely considered.

Numerous experiences show that obstacles and changes in the social and cultural environment generate modifications in neuronal structure. Perhaps the most spectacular example is that from years ago of the so-called wild children, together with cases of cruel imprisonment and deprivation of contact with other human beings. Even though at one time they were viewed as humans in a pure

---

[11] Doupe *et al.*, "The song system: Neural circuits essential throughout life for vocal behavior and plasticity." Also see Álvarez Buylla and Lois, "Mecanismos de desarrollo y plasticidad del sistema nervioso central."

[12] Kennepohl, "Toward a cultural neuropsychology: An alternative view and preliminary model."

natural state, it is now obvious that the cognitive faculties of children growing up in such situations are deeply and sometimes permanently affected; they show signs of mental retardation and they lack linguistic skills. This seems to indicate that conditions of extreme deprivation modify certain neuronal structures. But beyond this phenomenon of brain plasticity one might ask if part of the modifications are due to the fact that some cerebral circuits remain incomplete and eventually become atrophied. This could mean that there are neuronal structures whose normal functioning depends on their managing to extend their circuits outside the brain.

It seems important to reflect here on the traditional duality that neuroscientists go back to: the internal and the external. It is usually based on a general consideration: in order to understand living organisms the definition of the boundary separating them from the outside is necessary. The organism's own structures are found within their limits and life is defined as the maintaining of internal states that identify an individual singularity. For Antonio Damasio the internal environment is a precursor of consciousness. Regulation of the internal state contrasts with the variability of the environment surrounding the organism. Even the amoeba, which has neither a brain nor a mind, "manages to keep the chemical profile of its internal milieu in balance while around it, in the environment external to it, all hell may be breaking loose." From these types of basic considerations, Damasio insists that consciousness "happens in the interior of an organism rather than in public, even though it is associated with a number of public manifestations." He is convinced that consciousness is an "inner sense," connecting with a tradition established by thinkers as diverse as Locke, Brentano, Kant, and William James.[13] I understand and support the neurologists' resistance to metaphysical ideas that do not accept that mental functions, including consciousness, are based on brain activity. For this reason they usually reject Cartesian dualism. However, drawing the limits of the brain is not as easy a task as might be thought.

Without a doubt the brain activity on which consciousness is based has a stable character and organizes the internal mental environment in such a way that it ensures coherence and continuity of the individual organism. This internal brain activity accumulates information about the external surroundings in memory. However, as Gerald Edelman and Giulio Tononi have pointed out, this memory does not have a representational character. Apparently there is no brain language that – like a computer – operates by means of representations that implicate a symbolic activity. There do not appear to be semantic codes in neuronal processes. The brain functions in a manner similar to the immune system: antibodies are not representations of dangerous antigens, even though

---

[13] Antonio Damasio, *The feeling of what happens*, pp. 136, 83 and 126.

they form part of an immunological memory. In the same way, an animal reacts to the particularities of its surroundings without its organism being a representation of the ecological niche because of that.[14] This niche is not a complicated chaos of information, but rather it functions in a certain way as a relatively stable code system. However, if environmental instability increases, the human way of survival consists of the connecting of certain non-representational internal circuits with highly codified and symbolic cultural circuits, with semantic representations and syntactic structures, and with powerful artificial memories.

It seems to me that the connection between internal neuronal circuits and external cultural processes helps us build a bridge between the brain and consciousness. In a fascinating discussion between Jean-Pierre Changeux and Paul Ricoeur, the latter stubbornly resists accepting the idea that neurobiology can find that bridge. In contrast, Changeux, the neurobiologist, does not accept setting *a priori* limits and is confident that his science will end up solving the mystery. However, it is Ricoeur, the philosopher, who makes a statement that opens new perspectives: "consciousness is not a closed place, about which I might wonder how something enters it from outside, because it is, now and always, outside of itself." Changeux accepts the notion but points out that it is difficult to give a serious experimental basis to the idea of being able to do away with the internal/external relation.[15]

It is possible that the solution to the problem would be found in a type of research that does not accept the categorical separation between the internal neuronal space and the external cultural circuits. To that end, in my interpretation, cognitive processes would have to be thought of as if they were a Klein bottle, where the inside is also the outside. But it is very difficult for this kind of research to advance, because many neuroscientists tend to be allergic to using discoveries made in the social and cultural sciences. Psychology, supposedly a communication bridge, actually obstructed contacts and, as Michael S. Gazzaniga says, has become a dead discipline. Hardline neuroscience only accepts linguistics, though it tends to strip it of its rich anthropological context. It is symptomatic that Gazzaniga needs to suppose the existence of a translating and interpreting neuronal apparatus located in the left cerebral cortex, in charge of creating the illusion of a coherent individual consciousness.[16] Is that not a new dualistic vision that has taken the old homunculus and substituted it with an interpreting mechanism?

---

[14] Edelman and Tononi, *A universe of consciousness: How matter becomes imagination*, p. 94.

[15] However, Changeux gives the example of the mirror neurons, a discovery that has already stimulated many studies and discussions and that I will refer to later on. Changeux and Ricoeur, *Ce qui nous fait penser: La nature et la règle*, pp. 137 and 141.

[16] Gazzaniga, *The mind's past*, pp. 24ff.

4   Is there an internal language?

An interpreting mechanism inside the brain that has the capacity to translate neuronal codes to cultural symbols (and vice versa) can be a very attractive idea. The best-known and most influential expression of this idea was formulated by Chomsky, who encouraged a search for the inborn neuronal circuits of a universal grammatical structure common to all humans. Many neuroscientists doubt the existence of such a linguistic structure in the nervous system. And if such mediating circuits do exist, they have yet to be found. This is a thorny problem, not only because of its intrinsic difficulty, but also because it has been contaminated by the old polemic about the relative weight of the cultural versus the natural in the configuration of consciousness. Language is obviously located in the neuronal space, as well as in the cultural dimension. Rather than polemicize about whether language is incorporated more in one of the two regions than the other, I believe it is necessary to study linguistic structures as a bridge joining the brain with culture. I do not think it is sufficient to prove that language and its context exert an important influence and that, thanks to plasticity, modify nerve circuits. Nor is it enough to establish that inborn neuronal circuits leave their mark on language structure and its social environment. I prefer instead to explore the possibility that language forms a part of exocerebral networks that, as such, are not exactly inside the brain, but are not an independent phenomenon disconnected from the nerve circuits either.

Let us start from a concrete example. Research has demonstrated that there are different patterns of brain activity that separate semantic processes from grammatical systems. Through the study of event-related potentials (ERPs),[1] it has been determined that the use of nouns and verbs (lexical and semantic information) provokes a particular brain activity that implicates a greater activation of the systems located in the posterior temporal and parietal lobes. In contrast, the use of prepositions and conjunctions (grammatical and syntactic information) activates frontal parietal regions of the left hemisphere of the brain. On the other hand, different activation patterns that are dependent on whether

---

[1] Voltage fluctuations in the electroencephalogram in response to a controlled stimulus.

images transmitted by the retina of the eye come from the center or periphery of the visual field have also been observed. This research indicates the presence of two plasticity patterns in relation to visual and linguistic information processing in the brain. Systems that are sensitive to experience and learning throughout life are related to semantics, the topography of sensory maps, and the form of objects. In contrast, neuronal systems that are modifiable during early and limited periods of growth are related to grammar and the computation of changing dynamic relations among locations, objects, and events. As far as visual images are concerned, those that come from the center of the visual field (and that have to do with form) favor ventral pathways that project from the first visual area (V1), while those that come from the periphery (and are related to localization and movement) preferably use dorsal pathways.[2] This general hypothesis is supported by the known fact that the greatest plasticity for learning the structure of a second language takes place in childhood, while accumulation of vocabulary is possible throughout a lifetime.

Of course from this we cannot conclude that the syntactic-grammatical system is inborn, whereas the lexical-semantic system is culturally acquired, or that spacial images are not innate, while dynamic images are. It has been proved that different processes use relatively separate circuits and that each one of them is characterized by having different degrees and types of plasticity. Each system has a different dependency relation with respect to learning and social experience. Patricia Kuhl points out that we are facing two alternative interpretations. On the one hand, we can assume, along with Chomsky, that there is a genetically programmed neuronal development that implements learning processes, but whose development is not modified by experience. On the other hand, the second interpretation has a bidirectional character: brain development implements and propels learning, but it also propels the development of nerve circuits; this interpretation has its source in the ideas of Vygotsky. Kuhl leans toward the second interpretation and proposes that both the linguistic information input and the social interaction that take place during the first years of life are necessary and produce brain maps that alter perception.[3] The need to access linguistic information appears to be inborn, but the brain depends on the use of symbolic and logical processes that neuronal networks cannot process without resorting to cultural mechanisms. For example, the fixation of a spectrum of significant phonetic distinctions, which is characteristic of every language, is a process that takes place very early in childhood, before words are learned. But a clearly identified language center in the brain has not been located. Studies in people who have learned a second language later in life have shown that two distinct regions of the cortex are activated. Kuhl concludes

---

[2] Neville and Bavelier, "Specificity and plasticity in neurocognitive development in humans."
[3] Kuhl, "Language, mind and brain."

that later acquisition of a new language is difficult due to the fact that mental speech maps – drawn in the first language – are not compatible with the maps required by the second language, and so they are constructed in a different region. The most recent studies confirm the problem we are facing: there is no unified language area in the brain where linguistic signals are computed and processed. Different circuits are involved in language processing, and linguistic functions are not restricted to Broca's and Wernicke's areas.

And nevertheless, the brain is not a Tower of Babel. Language use reveals structured and stable brain activity. Where does this order come from? Is there an internal brain language that gives coherence to the connections between different areas of the central nervous system? It has been proved that when abnormal filtrations among different brain circuits occur, strange and revealing effects appear. Synesthesia is a condition in which different signals are crossed and mixed together. As such, a signal of touch produces a bitter flavor, a musical note when heard elicits the color blue, or certain numbers printed in black are seen as another color. The neurologist Vilayanur S. Ramachandran and researcher Edward Hubbard, who have studied this phenomenon, state that there is a genetic component that weaves connections in the brain between areas that are normally separated. Genetic mutation causes a communication excess among different brain maps: if the porosity is very extensive a synesthetic condition is created, but if it is not very wide, it simply stimulates a creative propensity toward finding links between concepts and ideas that have no apparent relation to one another. The authors of this research believe, and rightly so, that it is a condition that can help in understanding the origin of language. The emergence of symbolic and metaphoric association between visual and sound sensations in primitive hominids could have been an important lever in the formation of names for objects. A synesthete, for example, connects the number 5 with the experience of the color red. It is a spontaneous connection between a symbol and a sensation. It is interesting to note that many synesthetes do not see the color red when they read the Roman numeral V. In these cases it is not the concept of a number, but rather a visual grapheme that creates the color vision. There are other synesthetes that do respond to the numerical concept, which could be due to the precise place in the brain where the interconnection or the short circuit is produced.[4] We can assume that a primitive mutation could make a new connection between areas that were previously separate from one another, which in turn led to the emergence of symbolic and metaphoric relations. But the important thing is that one of the interconnected circuits has what could be called an open window to the social and cultural environment. What is new is that this window enables the

---

[4] Ramachandran and Hubbard, "Hearing colors, tasting shapes."

detection and use of external symbols as part of a process that represents signals of the environment through sensations. This brings to mind the intuition of Marshall McLuhan, who realized that mass media communication such as radio and television are "massive extensions of our central nervous system" that have "enveloped western man in a daily session of synesthesia."[5] In reality this synesthetic unifying force has been in operation for millennia but on a smaller scale.

Many neurologists contend that memory circuits do not have a representational character and that there is no language of thought. As I have pointed out, this is the position of Gerald Edelman and Giulio Tononi, who explain nonrepresentational memory with a metaphor: the memory system would be like a glacier that is warmed by the sun and melts into many streamlets that empty into a strong stream that in turn feeds a pond in a valley. Climatic cycle variations may change the stream configuration and form new ones. Even a new pond that is associated with the first can be created. The sequence is repeated with great stability, the same water flow descends each year even though it empties differently. Changes in temperature are similar to synaptic variations, and the stream systems are like the neuroanatomy. All of this takes place with no need for codes, symbols, or metaphors, nor is there a need for images or representations projected in the brain in such a way that they would be contemplated and deciphered by a mysterious spectator homunculus.[6]

This situation brings us face-to-face with the question of explaining the way in which neuronal circuits lacking symbols or representations can be connected with highly codified cultural circuits that are governed by symbolic, semantic, and syntactic networks. Even supposing that the brain functions according to yet undiscovered codes and symbols, we have to explain the way in which two distinct systems of apparently different nature communicate. And this takes us back to where we started: the idea of looking for a mediating and translating apparatus in the brain, capable of transforming external codes into chemical and electric signals. Regardless of whether or not this translating neuronal apparatus exists, I would like to underline the fact that there is a common aspect of mental operations related to symbols: at many moments of the process they turn to the external environment to obtain information and to confirm or process brain activity. Without a doubt, the brain is not a chaotic internal space, but it is important to point out that in a certain way the coherence and unity of conscious

[5] McLuhan, *Understanding media*, chapter 31.

[6] Edelman and Tononi, *A universe of consciousness*, p. 99. In contrast, Antonio Damasio says that the neural representations, which consist of biological modifications created by learning in a neuronal circuit, become images in our mind (*Descartes' error*, chapter 5). Neuron "firings" that are action potentials that depolarize the neurons are usually considered to be something like "the fundamental phoneme of the brain," to use Simón Brailowsky's expression (*Las sustancias de los sueños*, p. 54).

mental processes are provided by the exocerebrum, and in an outstanding way by linguistic structures that have become stabilized in the cultural environment over thousands of years.

I am not arguing in favor of the idea of the mind as a blank slate, a notion that is both uninteresting and unscientific.[7] Culture is not a blank slate or a blank page, either. I have emphasized the importance of plasticity in the nervous system in order to reflect on the fact that cultural environment is essential for the development of certain brain structures. This seems to indicate the possibility that there are also brain systems that are not very flexible and whose growth is determined by genetic factors, but that nevertheless depend on social experience and need cultural circuits in order to operate normally. In short, the question that arises here is the following: do neuronal correlates of language and consciousness exist? When Christof Koch and Francis Crick take on this question they maintain that the brain, in order to be conscious of an object, has to build a symbolic interpretation of the visual field on multiple levels. It is an explicit process – namely, a somewhat reduced group of neurons that employs a not very refined encoding process to represent a part of the visual field. Unlike Edelman, these researchers believe that there *are* representations in the brain circuits, and they propose a hypothesis: the neuronal correlate of consciousness must have access to explicitly encoded visual information and it is directly projected onto the planning stages of the brain associated with the frontal lobes and prefrontal cortex.[8] Crick and Koch consider that this neuronal correlate is the synchronized firing of neurons that symbolize the different attributes of the same visual object. More specifically, they would be periodic oscillations of different groups of neurons at a mean frequency of 40 cycles per second (40 Hertz). These oscillations had been registered in 1981 by two German research teams who thought they were the explanation for the way in which different groups of neurons bind together and correlate among each other to form a unified image of an object.[9]

It is an interesting hypothesis, but until now there have been no strong indications that these bonds coordinated by oscillations at 40 Hertz are actually a representational-type symbolic encoding action characteristic of a neuronal correlate of consciousness. The framework of this hypothesis is the image of a

---

[7] Those who still have an interest in this archaic theme can consult Steven Pinker's book, *The blank slate*. It is a very long tract criticizing a concept that is already like a building in ruins, and attempts to legitimize an alternative view through an effortless demolition.

[8] Koch and Crick, "Some thoughts on consciousness and neuroscience," p. 1291.

[9] See an intelligent panoramic explanation of this question in Francisco Javier Álvarez Leefmans' "La emergencia de la conciencia." Francis Crick presents his general vision of the problem in his book, *The astonishing hypothesis*, chapter 17. By 2002 Koch and Crick no longer believed that oscillations at 40 Hertz were "sufficient condition" for neuronal consciousness correlates ("A framework for consciousness").

nervous system seen as an immense network of wires connecting to neurons. Each neuron has a long ramification (axon) that conducts electric signals to a synapse that emits chemical signals through neurotransmitters to a receptive dendrite of the contiguous neuron. Neurobiologist R. Douglas Fields maintains that this landscape does not take into consideration the large brain mass made up of glial cells that tend to be thought of as the glue that supports the neurons, ensures their adequate chemical context, and isolates axons through myelin production to facilitate rapid signal conduction. But it is now known that glial cells are capable of communicating among one another and with neurons (through chemical, not electric, means) and can participate in the strengthening of synapses, a process that is typical of this form of plasticity that responds to learning experiences.[10] This new research is opening up an immense field, given that there are nine glial cells for every neuron in the brain. However, here too, the precise codes that regulate the chemical signals that are transmitted are not known.

The existence of an exocerebrum leads us to the hypothesis that brain circuits have the capacity to use symbolic resources – the signs and signals that are found in the environment – in their different conscious operations as if they were an extension of internal biological systems. Exocerebral circuits would substitute symbolic functions that the nervous system cannot perform. However, this does not imply that it is unnecessary to look for the electro-chemical codes through which the brain operates. In a certain way this extends the question of the search for the link that unifies the activity of various disperse neuronal sets in the brain in order to achieve the unified image of an object. Now the link between the brain and the exocerebrum must be looked for, and not reduced to the crude notion of an environment that emits signals or stimuli and a nervous system that provides access to information in order to process it and to instruct the body to act accordingly.

[10] Fields, "The other half of the brain."

5   Amputations and supputations

The external environment closest to the brain is the body itself. The senses of sight and hearing both receive a wealth of information proceeding from the extracorporeal world. In contrast, the motor and sensory maps of the cerebral cortex are connected to intracorporeal experiences. Each hemisphere of the brain contains maps of the opposite side of the body. These maps are very stable throughout life and they are similar in all individuals. However, accidents that involve the loss of an extremity or the interruption of the nerve flow coming from some part of the body provoke important modifications in the sensory and motor maps. Studies on monkeys have shown that each finger of the hand and different regions of the palm and back of the hand are drawn in a precise zone of the cortex in an order and arrangement similar to the extremity's form. If the third finger is amputated (or its nerve flow is segmented) the contiguous brain areas corresponding to the second and fourth digits will invade the third finger's space soon after. This modification is reversible if the nerve flow is restored. There is a good deal of information on the plastic adaptations in the cerebral cortex of different mammalian species when their extremities have been amputated: in all examples the corresponding areas respond to impulses that come from adjacent cortical zones, although sometimes some part that fails to receive body signals can remain silent. Added to this mysterious reorganization is an extraordinary discovery: the brain area corresponding to the paralyzed arm of a monkey is activated when the face, especially the chin and the jaw, is touched.[1] And so the following question comes to mind: why are regions of the cortex that correspond to a paralyzed or amputated part of the body inserted into a massive reorganization process of the brain map instead of remaining deactivated and silent? Why is there this singular expression of *horror vacui*? Researchers do not have an answer. And, as we shall see, the consequences of the reorganization that erases the empty silent spaces have strange and apparently undesirable effects. But if we go back to the idea that there are incomplete neuronal processes that require exocerebral circuits in order to function, perhaps this

---

[1] Pons, Garraghty, Ommaya, Kaas, Taub and Mishkin, "Massive cortical reorganization after sensory deafferentation in adult macaques."

peculiar aversion to emptiness is understandable. The neuronal groups that suddenly lose their functions try to become complete through their reconnection with other neighboring circuits.

The discovery of the extraordinary plasticity of the sensory and motor maps resulting from wounds and amputations attracted the attention of V. S. Ramachandran, who was interested in understanding the curious phantom limb phenomenon perceived by people who have suffered the amputation of an extremity.[2] He soon recognized in his patients what had been observed in experiments with macaque monkeys, rats, and other mammals: despite having lost an extremity they perceived its presence and even came to feel pain in the non-existent limb. A phantom hand was not an outlandish effect of psychic supputations or reckonings with no physiological base: that person actually felt his missing hand if his chin or forearm was touched. In fact, each finger of the amputated hand could be stimulated very precisely following the invisible drawing the researcher was discovering in the patient's face and forearm. Soon he discovered other cases in which the person had sensations in the phantom limb when other regions were stimulated: a woman felt her missing foot when she made love, another claimed to even have orgasms in her amputated foot, and a woman who had had a radical mastectomy experienced erotic sensations in her phantom nipples when her earlobes were stimulated. Ramachandran offers two possible explanations. It could be the growth of new sprouts or buds in the nerve fibers, but with this hypothesis it is not clear how the process can take place in an organized fashion. Another possibility is that there is an enormous redundancy of connections, an overabundance of unused links or links with no specific function that, like a reserve army, would enter into action when needed. According to this last hypothesis there would be inhibited connections between the cheek or the genitals and the zone of the cortex that is linked to the hand or foot. The inhibition would cease the moment the normal signal flow was interrupted.[3] But this does not explain the fact that reserve or inhibited connections are activated for no reason: why do we need to have an orgasm in a phantom foot? What is the purpose of feeling a tickling sensation in an amputated hand or suffering intense pain in a non-existent leg? In any case, whether new connections appear or existing ones become uninhibited there is an underlying tendency – genetically determined, I suppose – that does not allow certain neuronal groups to live in a condition of turned-off incompleteness. Circuits tend to be completed, even if in an aberrant way.

The best known cortical map is the one drawn by the neurosurgeon Wilder Penfield in the form of a homunculus lying down, with its head hanging over a

[2] Ramachandran and Blakeslee, *Phantoms in the brain*, chapter 2.
[3] Glial cells of the central nervous system that emit molecules inhibiting axon growth could have a function in these processes.

brain hemisphere and with its extremities represented in proportion to the size of the region of the motor cortex they are linked with: in the center there is an enormous hand with a huge thumb above which, going upward, is a tiny body stuck to a bigger foot with the genitals over the toes; in the other direction, going downward, is a tiny neck and a face with a very bulky mouth, large eyes, and a long tongue that is not on the face. Scientists do not only draw sensory maps related to movement. The sensations of heat, cold, and pain have their particular maps, as do the tactile signals. More than thirty maps related to the sense of sight have been depicted. The stability of these maps is sometimes altered by the dysfunction or interruption of certain circuits. That is when abnormal short circuits generating a complex feedback process are produced and different neuronal chains intervene. Ramachandran demonstrated the importance of visual circuits in the development and modification of phantasmal sensations. Through a system of mirrors he was even able to eliminate parts of a phantom arm, change its rigid position to a more comfortable one, and eliminate pain. Interested in defining corporeal identity and consciousness, he carried out various experiments in normal individuals to make them feel that the nose of another person, a plastic hand, a chair, or a table were part of their bodies, the same sensation someone driving a car has when he perceives the machine as an extension of his somatic identity. In Ramachandran's view, the body itself is a phantom that the brain has constructed merely for its convenience: the stable image that the individual has of her or his body, in which the self is anchored, is a transitory internal construction, a supputation that can be modified even through simple tricks.[4] I interpret this statement as the recognition of the presence of extracerebral networks that have at least two components: first, the organs and parts of the body that the nerves reach and, second, the material extension that the cultural environment provides. I believe that, in a strict sense, the exocerebrum only encompasses the second component, together with symbolic and linguistic networks. But experimentation with the first component – the somatic one – provides us with keys for understanding the mediations between the brain and its cultural environment, especially when the somatic counterpart has an immaterial and phantasmal character.

These phantasmal extensions of the body – are they the product of brain map modifications with no genetic cause or are they an effect of the spectral persistence of an inborn and genetically determined bodily image? Ramachandran answers this question by saying there is surely an interaction between both factors. I believe the fact must be emphasized that an anomalous sensory substitution is produced, whose peculiarities certainly may be due to modifications that are

---

[4] Ramachandran and Blakeslee, *Phantoms in the brain*, pp. 58–62.

relatively contingent on the map, but also to a powerful tendency to complete the absence and fill the void with the remains of an original bodily image.

We can understand that the relation between the brain and the external environment is similar to the one between the central nervous system and the peripheral extremities of the body. There are relatively stable neuronal maps that encode the particularities of our environment. Here, we come up against a problem indicated by some of the neurologists that I have mentioned before. In Jean-Pierre Changeux's concept, the problem lies in the fact that we live in an "unlabeled" universe that does not send us encoded messages. We project the categories that we create, with the help of the brain, onto a world with no destiny or meaning. The universe lacks categories, except, Changeux clarifies, those created by man. Here, the neurologist is answering a statement made by the philosopher Paul Ricoeur, who believes thinking of mental activity in terms of representation is a bad habit left over from Cartesian dualism. Changeux feels that representations are stabilized in our brain, obviously not like impressions in wax, but indirectly and after a process of selection that Edelman calls Darwinian.[5] Without a doubt, the ecological niche of a higher mammal is not a platonic world full of previous ideas, true propositions, and harmonies that some privileged beings – we humans – can decode. But neither is it a chaotic space without any rules. And the cultural environment especially, as Changeux recognizes, is without a doubt a world full of categories, labels, and symbols. How does the brain manage to encode, process, and map the cultural habitat?

Let us return for a moment to the links between the central nervous system and the hand (amputated or not). A question comes to mind: does the brain need a representation of the hand? Is the area of the cortex where we discover a kind of drawing of a macaque's hand a representation? I think not. I do not see why the brain would need a kind of photography of the hand, if it already has something better: the hand itself. The very complex sensorimotor feedback system that links the hand with the brain and that surely uses certain codes is something else. The truth is that we still cannot read the "synaptic hieroglyphics," as Changeux calls them, to be able to understand the precise operations that the brain performs when the hand moves or when pain is felt in the phantom leg that was amputated years before. But neuroscience is getting closer to the explanation, especially to the degree in which it has been moving away from the idea that the consciousness of having and moving a hand or of looking at a sunset implicates the existence of a small "I" that lives in the brain and contemplates the representations of the fingers and the back of the hand, or the color movie of the beautiful end of an afternoon.

[5] Changeux and Ricoeur, *Ce qui nous fait penser*, pp. 107–109.

The common ground at which those interested in cognitive neurobiology usually arrive is almost inevitable: how do we explain our individual experience when we perceive the color red? It is usually supposed that the experience of red is subjective and essentially private, a type of sensation that anglophone philosophers call *qualia* and that exemplifies the most difficult problem to solve: how to unify the first-person subjective experience of contemplating red with the third-person description of the scientist who defines the sensation as the activation of certain neuronal networks when a luminous ray of a determined wavelength enters the retina. In other words: what unifies the mind and the brain? Without a doubt, the category "red" does not exist in the universe. Neither does the category "arm." But these categories do exist in culture and in our language. They also appear in our brain map, although it is not certain that representations of the color red and the arm are there. Why do we need representations if we have access to both the member and the color thanks to the mediation of nerves and the retina? The fact that sensations do not come from objects that have an identifying card stuck to them ("this is red," "this is an arm") does not mean that these objects do not exist.

For Ramachandran the problem lies in the fact that we are facing two mutually unintelligible languages – the language of nerve impulses and the languages we speak. Therefore, I can only explain my sensation of red through speech, but the "experience" itself – he says – is lost in the translation.[6] Is it really lost? I do not think so. If it were lost, literature and art would not exist. The true problem to solve – an authentic mystery– is not the impossibility of translating subjective sensations expressed through speech into the neuronal codes that cross our brain. What we cannot explain is the strange fact that *yes* there is communication and therefore translation functions adequately.

A way to overcome the hurdle of non-communication, explains Ramachandran, is exemplified by the imaginary experiment that establishes a link between a person who is color-blind and one who is not. When the person with normal color vision is not able to communicate in words the experience of "red" to the person whose retina does not perceive color, an artificial nerve cable (made from nerve tissue cultures) joining the areas of the brain where color is processed is connected from one person to the other. In this way the information about color reaches the color-blind person without passing through the affected retina. This mental experiment, says Ramachandran, puts an end to the argument that there is an insurmountable barrier to the communication of *qualia*.[7] What

---

[6] Ramachandran and Blakeslee, *Phantoms in the brain*, p. 231.

[7] *Ibid.*, p. 233. Something rather similar to this experiment is carried out in subjects that are blind from birth through a transcranial magnetic stimulator that manages to activate certain areas of the cortical tissue with some degree of precision.

occurs in this imaginary experiment is that the normal person is transformed into a type of living prosthesis used by the person with achromatopsia. In my hypothesis, culture is what functions as the prosthesis, especially speech. It does not carry out a sensory replacement but instead it substitutes, through symbolic means, a communication that cannot take place by way of somatic mechanisms. In other words, there are links in culture that are equivalent to that artificial cable that conducts subjective experiences from one brain to another.

In 1928, the surrealist painter René Magritte made a mental experiment that should be of interest to neurobiologists. In his painting *The treachery of images* we see a pipe and under it the following inscription: "Ceci n'est pas une pipe." Magritte presents the image of a known object and the label declares that "this is not a pipe." There is a contradiction: our retina enables us to recognize a pipe, but our linguistic knowledge (if we know French) reveals the contrary. Apparently we are facing an unsolvable translation problem: upon looking at the painting we strongly feel the presence of a beautiful pipe, but a blunt message in another language warns us that we are mistaken. And nevertheless there *is* a possible translation. Although an inconsistency is produced between two different regions of the brain (the visual cortex in the occipital lobe and the areas of speech in the left hemisphere), any expert of modern western culture intuits the ironic paradox: obviously we do not see a pipe but rather a *representation* of one, and starting from this mind game we can perform many very sophisticated conceptual supputations on whether the linguistic message refers to the thing itself or to its image. Here the game can act as a reminder that images arrive coded and labeled by culture and that even the contradictions can contain messages that need to be deciphered. Magritte's painting confronts us with a doubt: what do we want with something that is not a pipe (it is its representation) if we can have the real thing and load it with tobacco and smoke it with pleasure? Why do we need art if we have daily life? Because representations and art enable us to translate what is apparently untranslatable.

It should be emphasized that an important, and perhaps fundamental, part of the translating apparatus is not found inside the brain, but rather right before our very eyes, functioning in the form of a vast cultural fan made up of languages, art, myths, artificial memories, mathematical reasoning, symbolic orders, literary tales, music, dance, classifying mechanisms, and kinship systems. All these aspects need to be explored from a neurobiological perspective in order to identify the precise exocerebral mechanisms that may be the key to the translating mediations between brain language and mental language and also help explain the phenomenon of self-consciousness. Speech is without a doubt one of the most important aspects of what I call the exocerebrum, but it is necessary to always take into account the context of the plastic symbols, rituals, beliefs, mnemotechnical signs, and mathematical systems that I have referred to. However, I would first like to put forward a theoretical reflection based on experiments that explore the language of apes.

A certain number of apes, whether captured in their natural habitat or born in captivity, find themselves in the laboratories of scientists interested in mental processes, neuronal networks, biocybernetics, the origin of language, or the study of different pathologies. It is not difficult to understand that this ape population, to some degree, undergoes more or less acute suffering, even if only for the fact of living outside its ecological niche. The world in which they live is filled with labels referring to strange categories and they find themselves forced to contemplate a highly ordered and articulated universe. Some of the luckier apes ended up in the laboratory of Sue Savage-Rumbaugh at the University of Georgia. There the chimpanzees not only were treated well, with affection and understanding, but they also had access to a particular prosthesis that enabled them to communicate with human beings; in addition, it substituted for the lack of an adequate vocal apparatus for speaking like humans because, among other things, chimpanzees cannot pronounce consonants. The situation of these apes can be compared with that of primitive humans moved to a strange and difficult environment, with the important difference that the *Homo sapiens* did not find adequate prostheses there, but had to create them instead. In contrast, the chimpanzees were trained to use electronic boards with keys marked with about one hundred symbols. When pushed, each key lit up and the corresponding symbol was simultaneously projected onto a screen. Something similar would have happened if our primitive ancestors had found an exocerebrum in the forest placed there by a benevolent alien from outer space, who would have taught them how to use it before returning to its planet. The apes in the laboratory, forced by the human environment and because of an electronic prosthesis, used brain resources that perhaps were not put to use in their natural environment.

In other laboratories, apes have been trained to use the sign language of the deaf. Surprisingly they have the ability to understand and ask for objects and food through the use of symbols and are capable of combining them and understanding that they represent actions or things. But the big surprise came when a young bonobo ape named Kanzi, who could understand some 150 words after the first 17 months of training, ended up constructing phrases on an electronic board with a primitive syntactic structure, was able to spontaneously acquire linguistic skills by means of social interaction with humans, as children do, and was capable of understanding complex sentences. Sue Savage-Rumbaugh has written a memorable book in which she relates her fascinating and touching search for linguistic abilities in chimpanzees. She presents a persuasive argument that chimpanzees have the basic neuronal machinery necessary for developing a primitive language and that human speech is not simply the effect of an inborn structure but rather the result of a plastic cognitive substrate that interacts with a social environment.[8] She is convinced that the human mind differs only in degree, but not qualitatively, from that of the apes. However, I find a qualitative difference: free chimpanzees in their natural state do not develop the complex type of language that they are capable of developing in captivity, surrounded by the human environment, and with access to a symbolic system that substitutes their inabilities. I believe this occurs not only due to the absence of an adequate culture, but also due to the fact that they do not undergo the effects of neuronal circuit dependency with respect to the linguistic prostheses that enable them to communicate. Chimpanzees in captivity depend on electronic boards to the degree that the human environment obliges them to. But it does not appear to be a neuronal dependency. They are capable of using a linguistic exocerebrum if it is given to them and they adapt to its use. But they do not have nervous circuits that are characterized by their incompleteness and their dependency on exocerebral circuits.

---

[8] Savage-Rumbaugh and Lewin, *Kanzi*, pp. 278–279.

6   The atrophied exocerebrum

We can take another path to search for signs of the exocerebrum within the central nervous system. In certain illnesses an accentuated atrophy is observed in the relation between the mind of an individual and his or her sociocultural environment. It has been known for a long time that lesions in the prefrontal region of the brain provoke antisocial and psychopathic behaviors. The celebrated case of Phineas Gage, the worker who had an iron bar go through his head in an accident in New England in 1848 injuring his frontal lobe, was the emblematic beginning of study on the subject: Mr. Gage went from being a kind and reasonable person to becoming unbearably irascible with a permanent blasphemous, obscene, undisciplined, and aggressive behavior.[1] Since then much information has been accumulated on the effects of prefrontal injuries. But now I wish to bring to my aid studies on antisocial people who have not suffered any injury. They are individuals who have been diagnosed by psychiatrists as having antisocial personality disorder: people characterized by continuous transgressive and violent behavior, constant aggressive irritability, and irresponsible indifference to the harm they inflict on others or on themselves.[2] We can assume that these disorders involve communication defects between internal neuronal circuits that have atrophied and circuits of the exocerebrum. This interpretation is confirmed by research results: people with antisocial personality disorder, according to images revealed by structural magnetic resonance, showed a significant reduction of prefrontal gray matter (but not white matter). Very importantly, two other groups were also analyzed in this research: drug addicts and schizophrenics, or people suffering from affective disorders. There was no reduction of gray matter observed in these groups, who are also people afflicted with pathologies causing serious social problems. The antisocial group showed an 11 percent reduction in gray matter in relation to the normal control group, a 14 percent reduction in relation to the drug addicts, and a 14.7 percent reduction in relation to the group with the other psychiatric

---

[1] See a summary of the case in Antonio Damasio's book, *Descartes' error*, chapter 1.
[2] Raine, Lencz, Bihrle, LaCasse and Colletti, "Reduced prefrontal gray matter and reduced autonomic activity in antisocial personality disorder."

disorders. Other aspects of the study showed that the deficit of prefrontal gray matter could not be attributed to psychosocial risk factors (such as low social class, divorced parents, family fights, criminality in the family environment, sexual abuse). In other words: the difficult social environment did not destroy their missing gray matter.

Autism is the mental imbalance that affects the connection of the brain with the sociocultural circuits in the most spectacular and disturbing way. It is interesting to recall that the classic text on autism published by Leo Kanner in 1943 describes these patients as "pre-hominid asocial animals," incapable of accepting or understanding changes in routine or in their environment, with no notion of the difference between "I" and "you," that develop good relations with objects and bad relations with people, and that have serious linguistic inabilities.[3] In other words, in my interpretation, they lack an exocerebrum. The cognitive ability of approximately 75 percent of autistics is significantly below average. Evidence seems to prove that autism has a biological origin with important genetic components.[4] It is important to mention that the disabilities of autistics do not arise from intellectual disability, given that a quarter of autistics do not have this condition. Beyond a low level of intellectual capacity, there is a nucleus of problems affecting all autistics: they lack the capacity to establish social relations, they have difficulty with verbal and non-verbal communication, and it is very difficult or impossible for them to imagine mental states or other people's intentions. Oliver Sacks has described the autistic condition of an intelligent professor at Colorado State University, Temple Grandin, with his characteristic depth and tenderness. She herself described her situation to Sacks: "A great part of the time I feel like an anthropologist on Mars."[5] She was referring to the lack of emotional empathy, her distance from the experience of others, and her difficulty in understanding behaviors and circumstances. She explains that to survive she had to accumulate a type of library in her memory where behaviors, experiences, and situations are catalogued in such a way that without feeling any empathy whatsoever, she is nevertheless capable of correlating events in order to understand and predict the behavior of that strange species of Martians that humans are for her. She feels that in her mind there are video tapes or computer discs that she can watch, like the proverbial Cartesian homunculus; but she cannot simply choose the instant of the movie she wants to see: her memory has to reproduce the entire scene. Sacks explains that general feelings of affection are not lacking in autistics, only those that have a relation "to complex human experiences, especially those of a social nature and perhaps those associated with them: esthetic, poetic, symbolic, etc."[6] Temple Grandin herself believes the visual parts of her

[3] Kanner, "Autistic disturbances of affective contact."
[4] Baron-Cohen, "The cognitive neuroscience of autism."
[5] Sacks, "An anthropologist on Mars."   [6] *Ibid.*, p. 288.

brain are overdeveloped, as well as those parts that enable her to simultaneously process a great amount of data. In contrast her verbal functions are underdeveloped, as are the areas of her brain related to sequence processing. She also believes the cause lies in her cerebellum, that it is a size smaller than normal, as magnetic resonance images have shown. The result seems to be that defects of certain parts of the brain are compensated for by extraordinary development of others.

There is evidence pointing to a symptomatic inverted correlation: autistic children have a serious incapacity in their psychological intuition for judging others, but their physicomechanical intuition is more refined than that in normal children of the same age. That is, they do not understand the behavior of people, but they understand the physical causality of objects.[7] They abhor personal contact, but machines fascinate them.

There is a strange and disturbing phenomenon accompanying autism: approximately 10 percent of autistics, who years ago were called "idiot savants," develop a kind of visual and acoustic memory hypertrophy such as extraordinary capacities for copying, reciting, or reproducing images, musical plays, and texts with great precision, but without understanding what they are doing. This syndrome generally occurs in individuals with very low levels of intelligence and affects males much more than females. Recent studies have demonstrated that these autistic savants have developed certain basic functions in the right brain hemisphere to an enormous degree, such as motor, visual, and non-symbolic activities. It seems like a kind of compensation for the dysfunctions of the left side, where the functions tied to logical sequences and linguistic symbolism are based. The result is that these autistic savants have almost incredible abilities in music, art, mathematics, calculus, and mechanics, but have serious inabilities in speech and language.[8] Research suggests that some kind of damage in the left hemisphere causes an abnormal activation of the right side, along with hypertrophy of the circuits tied to primitive forms of memory that lack semantic or cognitive content.

The connection with the symbolic substitution system is damaged or does not exist in the autistic, so that in certain cases – upon not being able to use cultural circuits – an expansion of the mechanical memory is produced that some researchers associate with striated cortical circuits (different from limbic cortical circuits linked to semantic memory).[9] In this type of living australopithecine, the neuronal circuits corresponding to language would be closed and complete and therefore would not look for connections with external prostheses. In a certain way it is like a terrible amputation, not of a body part, but of the channels that connect with the exocerebrum. The social and cultural

---

[7] Baron-Cohen, "The cognitive neuroscience of autism."
[8] Treffert and Wallace, "Island of genius." Also see Treffert's book, *Extraordinary people.*
[9] Squire and Knowlton, "The medial temporal lobe, the hippocampus, and the memory systems of the brain."

world of autistics is replaced by a memory that seems like a bottomless pit and by very unusual visual, auditory, and motor abilities. Replaced or substituted by a phantom exocerebrum with which they can make complex calculations in a few seconds, draw landscapes with extreme precision, and chronometrically and exactly mark time without the help of a watch. In Ramachandran's hypothesis a reorganization of the brain map has occurred.[10] I want to mention an example that has been intensely debated – the use of a prosthesis to connect an autistic person with her social environment. In 1991 a young autistic from California who could barely communicate verbally, Sue Rubin, was pushed to use a board with alphabetized keys to express herself, calling to mind the experience of the laboratory chimpanzees I described before. Apparently the use of this technique – called "facilitated communication" – enabled the autistic woman to come out of her isolation.[11] Having been considered intellectually disabled (with an IQ of 24) she ended up being, thanks to the board, an excellent high-school student, studying history at a university and living semi-independently at 26 years of age. At this age she still could not communicate through speech, but she wrote the script for a documentary film about her life, directed by Gerardine Wurzburg (*Autism is a World*, 2004, nominated for an Oscar). Is it possible that the electronic board substitutes the functional deficiencies of neuronal circuits that should communicate with her exocerebrum? It is an attractive idea, but there is still much to explore in the cases of autism treated through facilitated communication.

The fact that the malformation or reorganization of brain circuits is linked to more or less acute symptoms of sociocultural dysfunctionality in affected individuals confronts us with the old problem of correlations between the brain and consciousness, between the body and mind. It seems interesting to me to briefly discuss here three proposals that offer a solution to the famous problem. First I would like to cite the hypothesis of the psychologist Nicholas Humphrey.[12] His proposal is diametrically opposed to my interpretation: for him the mind is, in reality, a set of closed circuits and internal loops housed in the brain. It presupposes an evolutionary model by which, in an animal organism that changes habits and environment and therefore becomes more independent, the original responses to sensory signals stop being useful and having a real effect. The signals that conduct sensory responses form a short circuit before reaching

---

[10] Ramachandran and Blakeslee, *Phantoms in the brain*, p. 196.

[11] A critical description of this technique can be found in Smith and Belcher, "Facilitated communication and autism." Many researchers believe that the "facilitators" are those who induce the responses of the autistics that use boards. The case of Sue Rubin, however, seemed authentic to Dr. Margaret Bauman, autism specialist at Harvard Medical School.

[12] Humphrey, "How to solve the mind-body problem." This appeared in a monographic number of the *Journal of Consciousness Studies* focused on Humphrey's essay, with the commentaries of ten specialists.

the body's surface. Instead of reaching the sensory stimulus they arrive at points much nearer the nerve that provide access to the sensory signals, until there is a moment when the entire process is closed to the external world in an internal loop inside the brain. Although it seems like an explanation of the autistic phenomenon, according to Humphrey this is the origin of the mind: an interiorized process with a high degree of recursive interaction, a self-sufficient flow of signals that is self-made, that despite responding to an external stimulus, it has been converted into a circuit of signals that are referred to themselves. The mind, the same as consciousness, has ended up being a type of invagination of useless responses. However, as Stevan Harnad has shrewdly stated, Humphrey's solution has simply consisted of labeling the loops and closed circuits in the brain as "mental."[13] To put an end to the mind = brain equation, what he has done is merely declare that the mind is a brain activity and that the content of consciousness is made up of corporeal sensations. As Humphrey explains, the phantasm of the subjective sensation of pain can be equivalent to activity that is characteristic of a self-resonant state.

The autistic phenomenon confronts us with the need to determine if there are causal links between internal brain circuits and external cultural and social networks. Obviously the dysfunction of certain neuronal systems damages communication with the external world, which has dramatic effects on the behavior of an autistic. But something similar happens to a schizophrenic or a melancholic. The peculiar thing about autism is that there is a substantial interruption of the exocerebral circuits and so we can then ask ourselves if, at the same time, these external networks can have effects on the neuronal systems. Apparently exocerebral networks are a necessary part of certain neuronal circuits to such a degree that if they are amputated, internal tissues build a substitute phantasmal system. It can be inferred from Humphrey's thesis that in reality not only the substitutive hypertrophy of autism, but also consciousness, is a phantasmal sensation related to internal brain states. In contrast, I believe that normal consciousness is located in networks that connect neuronal circuits with exocerebral circuits.

Another psychologist has taken a very different path to explain how conscious experiences affect the brain. For Max Velmans the mind and the brain are ontologically complementary and mutually irreducible. His distinctive combination of ontological monism and epistemological dualism leads him to simply state that each individual has just one mental life, but two ways of knowing it: first-person "subjective" knowledge and third-person "scientific" knowledge. In this way Velmans can accept that conscious experiences are effective causes of brain states that do not violate the scientific principle of causal closure of the physical world and so therefore there is no metaphysical substance or spirit that

---

[13] Harnad, "Correlation vs. causality."

can influence it.[14] That is to say, what we consciously feel and think is not a mere epiphenomenon lacking causal powers, but rather one that has effects on what we really do. According to Velmans we have to live with the paradox of understanding the explanation of a third person in the chain of effects that a painful external stimulus produces in the central nervous system (the Cartesian *res cogitans*) and at the same time accept the presence of a subjective sensation of pain, a category that only exists in first person and that does not have an objective existence in the external physical world (the *res extensa*). And nevertheless, these two irreconcilable perspectives are related to the same sensation and the same information. Velmans' solution is that both perspectives are correct. Quite appropriately, it has been said that his solution to the problem of the relation between the brain and consciousness is purely verbal.[15] Velmans' idea renounces the study of causal connections that can exist between the mind and the brain. It simply refers us to the possibility already explored by researchers like Crick and Koch of finding consciousness-brain correlations, such as the case of synchronized neuronal firings at a 40 Hertz frequency discussed before.

I would like to make a third reflection, once again citing Gerald Edelman, the neurobiologist who has made important contributions to the study of the brain and has developed an attractive and complex theory about neuronal group selection.[16] Aware of the fact that it was necessary for him to approach the question of consciousness as causal, he has presented what he calls the "phenomenal transform" hypothesis. For Edelman a dynamic nucleus of neuronal interactions based on the thalamocortical system converts signals coming from the external world and the brain itself into a subjective consciousness capable of realizing qualitative distinctions based on semantic abilities. This phenomenal transform is not caused by the action of the nuclear neuronal process, but rather is a property of that activity, a process that accompanies and reflects underlying neuronal states upon which consciousness is based.[17] For Edelman, consciousness is an epiphenomenon that lacks causal power, but that reflects the causal capacity of the dynamic neuronal nucleus. The classic reference is T. H. Huxley's famous statement that consciousness is a collateral product of the body's functioning that has no power to modify that functioning, in the same way that the steam whistle accompanying the movement of a locomotive has no influence on its machinery. Huxley concludes that this is why we humans are conscious automatons. Edelman does not agree with the idea that humans are automatons, because his neuronal Darwinism and his explanation of the processes of selection do not let him think of the human body as a machine. However, the phenomenal transform is definitely like the locomotive's whistle or, to use the images of

---

[14]   Velmans, "How could conscious experiences affect brains?"
[15]   Gray, "It's time to move from philosophy to science."   [16]   Edelman, *Bright air, brilliant fire.*
[17]   Edelman, *Wider than the sky*, p.78.

William James, like the melody emanating from the strings of a harp that do not slow down or speed up their vibration, or like the shadow that goes alongside the traveler without influencing his steps.[18]

Edelman is aware of the fact that the link he proposes between the phenomenal transform and the neuronal substrate must be proved through experimentation. But he is certain that, given the close relation between both instances, we may speak as if consciousness were the cause of modifications in brain circuits even when knowing that such is not the case. Therefore, in order to explain the actual experience that enables qualities like the warmth of warm or the redness of red to be defined, it is sufficient to envision them as properties of a phenotype and to explain the basis of such distinctions. It does not seem like this explanation can help us get very far. Like Humphrey and Velmans, Edelman dodges the issue that autism and its antisocial behaviors have put before us: the cultural and social phenomena that qualify and give meaning to a large part of the sensations and perceptions arriving at the brain. We cannot avoid the problem of the influence of the sociocultural world on brain processes, no matter how much we proclaim that consciousness is an epiphenomenon, that it is actually a nervous process, or that it is the uncomfortable partner of an irreducible duality. Due to an almost mystical obsession with causal closure of the physical world, the cultural and social networks in which we live have remained outside the cloister.

It is obvious that cultural and social structures are a material phenomenon, but their reduction to the level of physical processes is completely useless and generates a brutal loss of the informative wealth by which we are able to understand sociocultural networks. The analytical degradation of these networks to their physical level means losing sight of what is essential: their structure. I bring this up simply to point out that the connection of brain circuits with sociocultural processes is not an operation that violates the causal closure of the physical world that scientists demand. It is not about inventing a meta-brain, but about studying the peculiarities of an exocerebrum.

An important consequence of a study of this kind is the need to understand that culture cannot be reduced to the set of socio-cognitive "abilities" that enables humans to manage symbolic systems, to identify with other persons, predict their behavior, and to learn and practice a way of conducting themselves characterized by social acts. Even though culture is based on certain abilities,

---

[18] See the citation of Huxley in William James' commentaries in chapter 3 of his *Principles of psychology*. In reality the whistle or melody can have causal power. If we think of them as signals that are transformed into symbols in a particular cultural system, we see that if a whistle does not sound, it can cause the locomotive to crash into a car at a railroad crossing and stop, and that if a melodic flow is inadequate, it can cause the harpist to be fired and also the silence of the harp. The epiphenomenon stops being one as soon as it integrates with a symbolic symbol capable of influencing the development and configuration of brain processes.

symbolic and institutional structures are not the sum of cognitive capacities of the brain. The widespread idea expressed by Tomasello that "all human cultural institutions rest on the biologically inherited socio-cognitive ability of all human individuals to create and use social conventions and symbols" is insufficient.[19] The problem is that this statement ends up being banal if it is not understood that there are complex social and symbolic systems between cognitive abilities and cultural institutions that are endowed with a logic of their own, with developmental rules and structures that cannot be reduced to individual abilities. The fact is that there are circuits in cultural and social phenomena that are found outside the brain and that cannot be explained by central nervous processes, by neuronal memory capacity, by inborn cognitive modules, or by brain abilities that function as what psychologists call a "theory of the mind" that allows us to recognize the intentions of others. Despite the fact that the brain houses more than 100 billion neurons and that these form a network of one quadrillion synaptic connections, cultural and social structures do not fit inside it: there is no way that the brain can absorb and contain in its interior any more than a small part of the sociocultural circuits. The brain, to refer to Emily Dickinson's celebrated poem, is vaster than the sky, deeper than the sea, and weighs as much as God; but human culture surpasses it by far.[20]

---

[19] Tomasello, *The cultural origins of human cognition*, p. 216.

[20] "The Brain – is wider than the Sky – / For – put them side by side – / The one the other will contain / With ease – and You – beside – / The Brain is deeper than the Sea – / For – hold them – Blue to Blue – / The one the other will absorb – / As Sponges – Buckets – do – / The Brain is just the weight of God – / For – Heft them – Pound for Pound – / And they will differ – if they do – / As Syllable from Sound –" Dickinson, *The Complete Poems* (poem 632).

7   The symbolic substitution system

I do not claim that the vast social and cultural structures are a giant exocere-brum, a colossal prosthesis composed of endless symbolic circuits. Such a lax definition loses explanatory strength and hurls us into the abyss of the common-place and the obvious. Nonetheless, it seems the immense vastness of culture does not contain all the secrets of its structure and evolution. The studies of anthropologists, historians, linguists, sociologists, and psychologists have con-stantly shown the need to turn to metasocial explanations in order to complete the interpretation of cultural phenomena. I am not referring only to the search for religious and metaphysical paths. The tendencies to look for answers in the social mentalities, the collective unconscious, archetypes, natural selection, genes, or the structure of the brain are more significant. In my opinion, these concerns are reactions to a real problem that is difficult to solve. There seems to me to be an incompleteness in sociocultural structures that is especially noto-rious in myths, symbolic language, visual imagery, or kinship relations that is similar to the incompleteness I believe exists in certain neuronal circuits. But the search for extracultural "causes" or "origins" has come up against many difficulties for creating an explanatory model capable of unifying biological and cultural structures. It would appear that we are facing worlds that are just as unconquerable as theological mysteries and secular realities tend to be. Perhaps it would be more creative to stop looking for a metacultural or extrasocial causality and instead confront the problem of deciphering a web of interactions that has its own dynamic: the network that joins the brain with the exocerebrum. To bolster these searches and reflections, I will make use of ideas developed by neurologists, biologists, and psychologists who have explored the world of culture.

Exocerebral circuits constitute a symbolic substitution system. This means they substitute certain brain functions by means of symbolic operations, which in turn, increase neuronal circuit potentialities. A simple example is the use of artificial memories, a primitive form of which is the simple accumulation and classification of objects that symbolize particular situations, persons, localiza-tions, relations, pacts, actions, intentions, or rituals that can be recorded at moments and in contexts that are not directly related to what is to be memorized.

An encoded collection of natural and artificial objects requires, of course, the capacity to give each one a name. Speech based on sounds that symbolize actions, objects, and persons is tied to the capacity to produce symbolic visual images that are expressed in many different types of paintings, statuettes, sculptures, and figures. To complete this minimal view of exocerebral resources, we can add the capacity to exchange visual and verbal signs and symbols, which is what propels mythological forms of imagination and enables kinship units and systems to be identified. I would venture to add the use of music (song and percussion) to interconnect embryonically ritual links between symbolized situations and emotional states. Thus the first anatomically modern men of 250 thousand years ago had a reduced exocerebral package made up of a few components: speech, kinship systems, visual imagery, music, dance, mythology, ritual, and artificial memory. Of course this exocerebral package relied on the abilities to produce and use primitive stone instruments (and undoubtedly tools made from perishable materials such as wood, which have not lasted).

Certainly, we can find examples in non-human animal species of communication, encoding, and memorization processes. However, what is peculiar to the human exocerebrum is that it substitutes functions that other animals carry out through non-symbolic processes. Animals exchange signs, which in some cases are movements of an action not completely carried out or interrupted, and they can analyze and memorize information proceeding from their environment. But we find hardly any signs of symbolic activity. The neurologist Elkhonon Goldberg, in his reflections on the relation of the frontal lobes to the civilized mind, says that the history of civilization has been characterized by a cognitive shift from the right brain hemisphere to the left, due to the accumulation of "cognitive templates" that are stored externally through cultural means and that are internalized by individuals during the act of learning, as if they were prefabricated modules.[1] In a way, these prefabricated cognitive templates that are accumulated extrasomatically are what I call a symbolic substitution system, although I prefer a more restricted and operational definition. These templates make the extraordinary capacity to store and transmit collective knowledge over a period of many generations possible.

But we need to go a step further and consider the possibility that some of these templates form part of a circuit that joins certain brain functions with symbolic systems, a circuit without which the cognitive network could not operate. Goldberg is inclined to think that cognitive routines are more closely linked to the left brain hemisphere and that it would be the one responsible for there being a connection with prefabricated cultural templates. In contrast, the right hemisphere would be linked to cognitive innovation. The question he poses is whether

[1] Goldberg, *The executive brain*, chapter 5.

there is a biological mechanism that regulates the balance between "conservatism" and "innovation." Goldberg's hypothesis is that the specific handedness of humans (only 10 percent of people are left-handed), could be a mechanism controlling the delicate balance between tradition and innovation. According to this speculation, the traditional cultural repression against left-handed individuals would reinforce conservative tendencies. Goldberg speculates even further: "is it possible that moral development involves the frontal cortex just as visual development involves occipital cortex and language development involves temporal cortex?"[2] This idea is based on a previous supposition: that the main flow of this involvement goes from the cerebral cortex to morality, vision, and language. Therefore he asks whether the frontal cortex contains the taxonomy of all moral actions and sanctionable behavior. If we wish to advance, the question should be inverted: is it possible that the moral taxonomy contained in culture is necessary for the development of the cortex? The moral agnosia that could occur due to prefrontal cortex injury would not stem from the fact that the moral compartments of the brain were ruined but rather that – as in antisocial personality behavior – the circuits that communicate with the exocerebrum, the place where complex taxonomies are kept that cannot be stored in the central nervous system, would be damaged. Goldberg's speculative hypotheses would be even more stimulating if we were to think in terms of bidirectional flows between the cerebral cortex and external cognitive circuits.

When Goldberg tackles the subject of self-awareness he asks if the prefrontal cortex is capable of differentiation between self and non-self, of integrating information about the internal environment of the organism with data proceeding from the external world. Although Goldberg believes that this cortex is the only part of the brain endowed with the neural mechanisms capable of integrating the two sources of information, he relies on the hypothesis of the psychologist Julian Jaynes to suggest that consciousness of the self emerged late in history, perhaps only two thousand years before the Christian era. According to Jaynes, before the advent of this self-consciousness there was a double brain, different from the brain we have today. The functions characteristic of speech in the brain of today's humans are located in the left hemisphere: the supplementary motor cortex in the frontal lobe, Broca's area in the inferior part of the same lobe, and Wernicke's area in the posterior temporal lobe. Jaynes proposes that before the appearance of self-consciousness, the area of the right temporal lobe corresponding to Wernicke's area was active and organized hallucinatory experiences that enabled people to hear the voices of gods. For thousands of years, this peculiar "bicameral" mind prevented the development of self-consciousness because individuals were incapable of distinguishing

---

[2] *Ibid.*, chapter 9.

between self and non-self. Jaynes believes indications of the incapacity to distinguish the internal representation of other people from the presence of real individuals can be found in the early history of humanity, along with the impossibility of identifying voices emanating from the right hemisphere as being internal self-hallucinations, and so they are taken as divine, magical, and religious expressions.

For Jaynes, the *Iliad* of the eighth century BCE represents a bicameral epoch in which humans lacked subjective consciousness: with neither soul nor will, they were noble automatons manipulated by the gods. The mind was divided into an executive part and a dominated part: the first was the hallucinated voice of the divinity that, from the right hemisphere, propelled human activity and the second was the human who, with the left hemisphere, accepted the orders. None of these parts of the brain were conscious. Jaynes' line of argument is not convincing, because it reduces cultural manifestations to a narrow and lineal psychological interpretation. Many of the cultural manifestations that he considers to be typical of the bicameral mentality are, from my point of view, characteristics of the exocerebrum: mythic beliefs, music, oracles, religious hallucinations, possessed states, ritual phantasmagoria, and other similar forms of primitive or ancient religiosity. What Jaynes overlooks is the profoundly symbolic character of these cultural phenomena that are so embedded in analogous, allegoric, and metaphoric processes, as is speech, which he considers to be a separate process (belonging to the left hemisphere) linked to self-consciousness. The bicameral mind thesis would seem to indicate that biological evolution of the brain continued up until very recent times and that even today we could find individuals with archaic bicameral brain characteristics. Or as Goldberg says, it has to be accepted that self-consciousness cannot develop through biological evolution of the frontal lobes alone – cultural function is also necessary in order for that to take place.[3] I believe this is an adequate alternative, not only because of the immense accumulative capacity of cultural processes, but also because, as symbolic circuits, they complete the brain functions that stimulate the development of self-consciousness. The conclusions arrived at about the predominance of a divided brain and a bicameral mind based on the study of the *Iliad* and of ancient Mycenaean, Mesopotamian, Egyptian, Mayan, and Incan cultures, seem to me to be a forced psychological operation to prove the thesis that the emergence of self-consciousness is a recent phenomenon in human history. It assumes something that is not proved: total control of culture from brain command centers. Social and cultural structures appear as mere instruments of brain activity, lacking autonomy, and mere reflections of neuronal network capabilities.

[3] *Ibid.*, chapter 7. See Jaynes, *The origin of consciousness in the breakdown of the bicameral mind.*

The idea that biological evolution, based on natural selection, is insufficient for explaining the emergence of consciousness is not new. First of all, the great naturalist and anthropologist Alfred Russell Wallace should be mentioned, who together with Darwin discovered the principles of evolution by natural selection. Although these two scientists maintained very similar opinions, they disagreed precisely on the subject of the emergence of a brain capable of generating a complex and advanced consciousness in humans. Unlike Darwin, Wallace did not believe that the processes of natural selection could explain the emergence of the sophisticated expressions of consciousness characteristic of a biologically modern brain. According to Wallace, in order for this process to have emerged, the appearance of new causes linked to cultural processes was necessary. Wallace followed strictly scientific reasoning when he accepted that, once language and culture had intervened, human evolution would acquire Lamarckian forms, when the inheritance of acquired characteristics through extrasomatic means appeared. It is true that Wallace added some spiritualist hues to his theory to explain the mysterious emergence of the amazing capacities that led man to develop the mathematical, artistic, and musical abilities characteristic of the most advanced civilizations. He believed that only the intervention of invisible spiritual powers could drive the marvelous capacities of man: the "progress from the inorganic world of matter and motion up to man," he wrote, "point clearly to an unseen universe, to a world of spirit – to which the world of matter is altogether subordinate."[4] However, as Loren Eiseley has pointed out, the original formulation of the ideas that recognize the fundamental role of culture had nothing to do with his religious beliefs.[5] Ramachandran recovers the essential aspect of Wallace's idea: the discovery that there is a symbiosis between the brain and culture. Ramachandran affirms that both are as independent as the nucleated cell and its mitochondria or the naked hermit crab and its shell.[6] Another neurologist, Llinás, in his very stimulating book on consciousness, reminds us of that evolutionist hypothesis according to which vertebrates can be seen as inside-out crustaceans, with their skeleton on the inside and their flesh on the outside. He says that this does not happen with the brain, which is like a crab, covered by an exoskeleton.[7] But something takes place that is similar to what happens when hermit crabs look for an artificial exoskeleton in the empty shell of a snail in order to protect their nudity, like Diogenes. Comparably, outside the fragile cranium that hides it, the soft human brain flesh has searched for an artificial exocerebrum, exposed to the elements, that provides it with a solid symbolic support structure.

I have presented this back-and-forth between the evolutionary discussions of the nineteenth century and more modern neurological concepts in an effort to strongly emphasize the importance of studying the links between the brain and

---

[4] Wallace, "Darwinism applied to men," p. 476.   [5] Eiseley, *Darwin's century*, p. 296.
[6] Ramachandran and Blakeslee, *Phantoms in the brain*, p. 190.   [7] Llinás, *I of the vortex*, p. 4.

culture. Now I wish to discuss a concrete proposal that attempts to explain these connections. The zoologist Richard Dawkins has presented an argument analogous to that of Wallace: to understand the evolution of modern man we must discard the idea of the gene as the sole base for understanding that evolution. Cultural transmission is not explained by genetic processes of selection. According to Dawkins, there are units of cultural transmission, similar to genes, capable of propagating themselves by jumping from one brain to another, through an imitation mechanism that produces replicas. These units that are able to make copies of themselves were named memes. Dawkins proposes the existence of a unit of information (the meme) and a mechanism that produces its transmission (imitation). The meme is not a metaphor, but rather a particular structure of the nervous system of all individuals. Imitation takes place because the meme has the ability to survive as a result of the strong psychological attraction it produces in brains. Like Wallace (whom he does not cite), Dawkins maintains that the moment the conditions under which a new replicator can make copies of itself appear, a different type of evolution begins that no longer depends on the old mechanisms of genetic selection, responsible for having created brains, and which are something like the fertile primeval soup in which the first memes were born.[8]

The most serious problem confronting this theory is its total inability to identify the meme as the smallest unit capable of reliably and creatively replicating itself.[9] It is possible that *Don Quixote*, the Christian God, a catchy tune, a style of shoes, an infinitesimal calculation, the habit of hijacking airplanes, the myth of the wild man, a technique for producing bricks, the wheel, or the idea of evolution can each be this mimetic unit. Whatever idea or thing that manages to survive is a meme. As such, all the explanatory power is eliminated from this concept and it ends up being a simple banality referring to processes of cultural imitation and transmission. In reality this theory does not attempt to explain the reasons why certain ideas or practices survive, by studying their usefulness, their advantages, their location in a group, and other causes, because the search has been inverted: survival of the meme is not explained by its function, but rather by the fact that its replica benefits the same replicating unit.[10] This is why so-called memetics has not produced a single worthwhile analysis of culture.[11]

Nevertheless, we may ask ourselves if the meme hypothesis can explain some brain functions. From Dawkins' ideas, there are proposals that suggest a neuronal basis for memes: imitation and learning would produce a "warming" effect in groups of neurons resulting in greater firing susceptibility and would be the

---

[8] Dawkins, *The selfish gene*, pp. 191–194.   [9] Dennett, *Consciousness explained*, p. 201.
[10] Blackmore, *The meme machine*, p. 27.
[11] Kuper, "If memes are the answer, what is the question?"

basis for the signals that phenotypically express the meme.[12] The anthropologist Robert Aunger has proposed something similar: a small neuronal group (about one hundred neurons) would produce a back-up copy of the information it holds. The group would share a synaptic state of readiness for joint firing: this "state of alert" of the group of neurons capable of creating copies would be a meme. The series of electrical discharges of these groups form packages (he calls them trions) that are capable of moving about the brain, influencing mental events, and directing the organism's behavior. These trions can escape from the brain by inducing their hosts to translate them into new codes, through gestures and words, and thus spread themselves throughout the external environment.[13] Aunger defines the neuromeme as: "a configuration in one node of a neuronal network that is able to induce the replication of its state in other nodes."[14] The problem with these hypotheses is that they look for the neuronal substrate of a minimal unit of cultural transmission that has only been able to be very vaguely defined. In addition, there is nothing that proves that the neuronal group that produces synchronized discharges is more a support of the meme than it is a consciousness correlate or the representation of an image.

The philosopher Daniel Dennett has enthusiastically taken up the meme theory again and with his exuberant reflections has without a doubt stimulated the search for cultural processes linked to consciousness. When he speculates about the mechanisms that propel cultural evolution and the transmission of its products, he points out the importance brain plasticity must have had for our primitive ancestors in installing a program that regulates the habits of acquis-ition sharing. He suggests that the first hominids, now endowed with a rudi-mentary language, lacked the connections among brain areas that would permit cultural transmission program operation. Under these circumstances, individ-uals would have put self-stimulation systems of the missing connections into use, through speaking out loud, so that the vocalized information would be transmitted from the emitting brain sector to another area of the nervous system that auditorily received it. It would be as if there were a radio trans-mission generating virtual external wiring between two internally cut-off regions of the brain. Dennett suggests that this auditory self-stimulation must have stimulated new internal neuronal connections. In this way the entrance and exit pathways were built for the vehicles of language that were rapidly contami-nated by these parasites that are memes.[15] It seems more interesting to me to propose the opposite hypothesis: brain areas are *not* stimulated to build internal

---

[12] Delius, "The nature of culture."   [13] Aunger, "Culture vultures."
[14] Aunger, *The electric meme.*
[15] Dennett, *Consciousness explained*, pp. 193–194, 197 and 200. In an earlier work, *Sweet dreams*, Dennett seems to have forgotten cultural networks, keeping himself trapped in the tiring philosophical discussion with those who stubbornly insist on assuming that consciousness is a mystery beyond the reach of scientific research. A sharp and creative critique of Dennett's theory

communication channels since the external circuits function more efficiently and are capable of growing and spreading very rapidly. Perhaps Dennett does not contemplate this possibility due to the extensive obsession of finding all the answers to the question of consciousness *within* the central nervous system.

I believe that external circuits that communicate the zones of speech with those of hearing – to which we can add the external connections between the motor regions controlling the hand that draws, engraves, or paints, and the visual centers – form collective networks shared by the members of the human community. These peculiar self-stimulating connections are manifested in rich symbolic activity that is also charged with emotionality, music, ritual dance, artistic creation, verbal communication, memory that is accumulated by means of symbols or myths, information exchange, and support within extensive and well-structured family groups. This exocerebral nucleus most certainly includes mimetic and imitative capacities, but its complex symbolic network loses meaning if it is reduced to the action of memetic machinery that supposedly functions like a genetic machine.

can be found in Merlin Donald's book *A mind so rare*. He develops a very interesting inter-pretation of the links between culture and the brain. See also his previous book *Origins of the modern mind*. I find my hypothesis very close to his view on the development of hybrid minds. Donald has brilliantly surpassed previous ideas strongly influenced by the modular theory and by computational models.

Not only have some neurologists wanted to reveal the mystery of consciousness, but they have also attempted to discover the secrets of genius. The idea that the answer to the enigmas of consciousness must be locked inside the heads of history's most brilliant personalities has translated into an extreme curiosity on the part of certain scientists (and not a few charlatans) to carry out studies directly on the brains of geniuses. Slices of Albert Einstein's brain were given out to various scientists by the pathologist who performed his autopsy. This man kept the thinking organ of the great physicist in a jar for forty years. Close to the end of his life he decided to turn over what was left of it to the genius's granddaughter and so he traveled across the United States by car with the mortal remains. The neurologist Marian Diamond, of the University of California, examined some slices and could only determine that there was a large concentration of glial cells in the area of association (area 39 of the left hemisphere) of Einstein's brain that was greater than in other sections.[1] Apart from that, neither she nor any of the others could find the secret of genius. Of course there had been previous cases of great thinkers whose brains ended up in scientists' laboratories, such as the mathematicians Carl Friedrich Gauss and Sonja Kovaleski. Another famous brain that was the subject of detailed study was that of Lenin. Oskar Vogt, an important German neurologist, was hired by the Soviet government to discover the unique and extraordinary nature of the brain of the great leader of the October Revolution. Vogt, in his laboratory in Berlin, had developed refined techniques for cutting the brain into seriated sections for their study. This physician was looking for relations between mental processes and what he called the "architectonics" of the brain. Korbinian Brodmann carried out his studies of mammalian cerebral cortex cytoarchitecture in Vogt's laboratory, culminating in 1909 in the famous monograph that established fifty-two cortical areas. For two and a half years (between 1925 and 1927) in his Moscow laboratory, Vogt dedicated himself to slicing Lenin's entire brain into tens of thousands of sections that were meticulously mounted and

---

[1] Diamond *et al.*, "On the brain of a scientist." See also Paterniti, *Driving Mr. Albert*.

stained for their study. He observed that the third layer of pyramidal neurons of
the Leninist cortex were especially numerous and large. Vogt felt certain that the
great revolutionary had been born with these large nerve cells and that their size
was not a compensation (as perhaps we would expect) caused by the consequent
brain damage of a disease.[2] It appears that the scientists of that time who were
familiar with Vogt's report, published in 1929, were somewhat perplexed.

Of course, neuroscientists would prefer to put their instruments into a live
human brain, if they were able to do so without producing damage. But such an
intrusion is possible only on those few occasions when a surgical operation is
indispensible. Thus, neurologists who have perhaps dreamt of directly scruti-
nizing the brain tissue of geniuses have had to be content with opening the heads
of far less intelligent beings. But what they have found there is much more
interesting and revealing than what was found in the dead brains of Einstein and
Lenin. One of the most important events that took place during the so-called
decade of the brain was the discovery of mirror neurons in the frontal lobes of
monkeys by Giacomo Rizzolatti and his collaborators in 1996.[3] This discovery
opens up new scientific perspectives for understanding human brain evolution,
language emergence, and the mechanisms of consciousness. The finding is
apparently very simple: mirror neurons are visual and motor cells, originally
detected in the premotor ventral cortex of monkeys (area F5) that have the
particular characteristic of being activated when the animal performs an action
(such as grabbing an object), as well as when it watches another individual
(including humans) perform a similar action. The mirror neuron system is
possibly the neuronal basis of social forms of recognition and of understanding
the actions of other individuals. It should be emphasized that area F5 of the
monkey is homologous to Broca's area in humans. Monkeys recognize actions
performed by others because the neuronal activation pattern that is produced in
the prefrontal areas is similar to the pattern that is internally generated to
produce these same actions. This implicates the existence of a kind of "semantics" inscribed in the motor neurons that are capable of "representing" an action.
As can be seen, it is a specular circuit that recognizes acts in the social environment through neurons whose motor action is inhibited so that the action the
individual is contemplating is not set off. But they are the same neurons that, if
necessary, set the body in motion to perform an observed action (such as pull,
push, or grab objects). It is also necessary to add that these mirror neurons are
not activated (or if they are, it is minimal) if the action of the hand only imitates
the movement of taking an object when there is no object there. Neither are they
activated if the object is pushed with an instrument and not with the hand.

[2] Bentivoglio, "Cortical structure and mental skills."
[3] Rizzolatti, Fadiga, and Gallese, "Premotor cortex and the recognition of the motor actions."

However, even though it seems that we are dealing with a neuronal circuit linked to imitation, as far as is known, monkeys lack mimetic abilities.

There are solid indications that a system of mirror neurons also functions in the left hemisphere of the human brain. One study registered an increase – produced by motor impulses – in the potential of the muscles involved in an observed action.[4] Other studies indicate the existence of a specular recognition system: the observation of the act of taking an object activated the superior temporal sulcus, the inferior parietal lobe (area 40), and the inferior frontal gyrus (area 45 or Broca's area).[5] In the monkey brain, the mirror neuron system also involves a triangular connection formed by the superior temporal sulcus (through which visual signals possibly enter), the PF area in the inferior parietal lobe, and area F5 of the ventral precortical lobe.[6] These last two areas are homologous to Broca's area and area 40 in the human brain.

The hypothesis that has emerged postulates that the mirror neuron system observed in monkeys, in which motor functions not only control action but also represent it, may be the origin of a human representation system specialized in processing social information.[7] In other words, a rigid and encapsulated system capable of efficiently controlling the organism's relation with its environment would have been transformed into a flexible and open system capable of managing symbolic information proceeding from a rich and ever-changing multicultural environment. Rizzolatti and Arbib believe there was a progressive evolution of the mirror neuron system that would have produced the emergence of Broca's area from a precursory area similar to the monkey area F5, an area that already had mirror-like properties.[8] Thus, mimetic capacities, a hand and facial gesture sign system, and finally a symbolic vocalization system would have emerged. Through a gradual process of natural selection, first, mimetic capacity would have emerged, after which an encoded system of hand and gesticulation signs would have developed, to finally make way for the symbolic vocalization system that is speech. Human language would have evolved from a

---

[4] Fadiga *et al.*, "Motor facilitation during action observation."
[5] Rizzolatti and Arbib, "Language within our grasp."
[6] Fogassi and Gallese, "The neural correlates of action understanding in non-human primates."
[7] The social function of mirror neurons appears to be confirmed in a study carried out by Ramachandran and his colleagues. They observed that in humans there is a suppression of electroencephalographic mu waves when normal individuals move one of their hands or watch someone else move it. However, in autistics mu wave block occurs when they voluntarily move one of their hands, but not when someone else moves it. This seems to indicate that autistics suffer abnormalities in their mirror neuron system. Ramachandran, *A brief tour of human consciousness*, p. 119, n. 6. See a critical review of the theories that support the idea that mirror neurons are the basis of action understanding in Hickok, "Eight problems for the mirror neuron theory of action understanding in monkeys and humans."
[8] Rizzolatti and Arbib, "Language within our grasp."

basic mechanism that originally was not linked to communication, but rather to the capacity to recognize actions.

The hypothesis seems quite reasonable. Modifications of circuits made up of mirror neurons would now not only have enabled connecting with fixed and stereotyped hand movements of other individuals, but also with a flexible and creative social and cultural communication system made up of encoded signs, signals, and sounds. The advantages for primates endowed with these abilities are obvious and may have been a determining factor in the process of natural selection that opened the door for the evolution of anatomically and cerebrally modern man.

What triggered the changes in the primitive mirror neuron system? What stimulated the new uses for this neuronal structure? If we stop to consider the interpretations of those who have discovered mirror neurons, we can figure out some of the answers. An essential element is the fact that the registering of an act is accompanied by a series of mechanisms that impede the observer from initiating mimetic behavior that reproduces the contemplated action. There are inhibition processes in the spinal cord that selectively block motor neurons that could copy the observed action. However, on occasion the motor system allows a "brief prefix" of the intended action. The other individual who is carrying out the action would supposedly recognize this prefix and understand that the rapid, cut-off movement signified an intention. At the same time the observer would realize that his involuntary reaction affects the actor. At this point, the observer would have to have the capacity to control his mirror neuron system for the purpose of voluntarily emitting a signal. According to Rizzolatti and Arbib this embryonic dialogue would be the nucleus of language. However, this development seems to contradict the peculiarities of the mirror neurons themselves as they are observed in monkeys: these nerve cells are not activated if the object of action is not present. What would be the reason for this activation if the object were not there? It would have to be assumed that there was a mutation that allowed voluntary control of the inhibition mechanism, along with the consequent ability to perform hand signs. This hypothesis leads us to suppose the existence of a continuous flow of mutations that would gradually be leading the first humans from hand sign to gesture, and from gesture to phonemic vocalizations.

If we consider my hypothesis of the exocerebrum, perhaps we would reach a somewhat different explanation. We would have to begin from the opposite supposition: the inhibition and difficulty in copying the movement of others, already mentioned above, would be a condition added to the series of growing obstacles for recognizing the environment. It is true that the human mirror neuron system functions differently from that of monkeys. In monkeys the system is not the basis of understanding or of speech or even of intentional imitation. In contrast, in humans the system is not encapsulated. Not only is it a localized brain circuit, but it is also part of the flexible structure that enables speech.[9] At a certain moment, a significant change in the neuronal system of the first humans must have occurred that caused a large increase of mirror neurons, opened the system, and connected it to areas of the brain related to vocal articulation and signal processing. As a metaphoric image, let us suppose there is a human being that discovers a new potential: upon witnessing the act of another individual, it can pronounce syllables associated with the movement it sees. Here, we would have an example of a typical sensory substitution system. The inherent difficulties of the encapsulated mirror neuron system would be overcome by means of a circuit that would substitute sensory information input with the capacity to accept and process symbolic information. Specialists who look for mechanisms for helping the blind assert that, until now, the most successful sensory substitution system is that of Braille. They suggest that reading written signs may be thought of as the first sensory substitution system.[10] To my way of thinking, and using the same logic, the first sensory substitution system in reality was speech, even though in this case – unlike writing – there would be a genetically conditioned neuronal substrate. Syllabic sounds that represent acts and objects artificially substitute the sensory functions of recognition and interpretation that do not efficiently operate except within certain limits. If the action or object is not visible or has a new appearance that disguises it, the sensory system is incapable of interpreting the situation. But the articulated voice of another individual can symbolically signal the existence of the act or object that for some reason the senses cannot recognize (it has been destroyed or hidden, for example). As Rizzolatti has pointed out, the basis of this new capacity is the fact that, before the emergence of language, the precursor of Broca's area was endowed with a mechanism for recognizing actions carried out by others.

These discoveries question the Chomskyan theory of a universal grammar emanating from a single mental organ that mysteriously appeared at some point in time during the evolutionary process. The basis of speech is not a specific module, but rather it would have evolved from different neuronal structures that originally had no relation to communication mechanisms. A formalistic interpretation of language that greatly emphasizes syntactic structures to the detriment of semantic, metaphoric, and symbolic functions lends support to the idea that there is a genetically determined neuronal device for speech. It has its roots in the postulate that there is an inscribed universal grammar in the brain that upon connecting with the social environment, triggers and generates the development of different languages in children, all constructed from the same

---

[9] Stamenov, "Some features that make mirror neurons and human language faculty unique."
[10] Bach-y-Rita and Kercel, "Sensory substitution and the human-machine interface."

syntactic model. Many neuroscientists find this idea as sterile as the old Cartesian interpretation.[11]

It is best not to fall into the temptation of seeing speech-related neurological circuits as the headquarters of programs independent from the outside world, capable of applying abstract and formal syntactic rules to information that is filled with a high sentimental, semantic, and symbolic content proceeding from the social and cultural environment. In reality they are continuous circuits that connect the internal world with the external universe. Of course these circuits exist in all animals that establish a relation network with the ecological niche in which they live. For example, the act of walking does not implicate the operation of a cybernetic-type input/output information circuit, incorporated in a process of external data recognition which reveals that the ground is relatively even and that interacting with it involves the law of gravity. It is not an information circuit with which out-going instructions that govern leg movement and other physiological mechanisms can be given, as could be the case with a robot programmed to move about on the surface of Mars. The fact is that the motor and neuronal circuits operate under the supposition (unconscious) that gravity exists and that, to a certain degree, the ground is level. It is the operation of circuits that continuously interact with an environment that has been internalized. Conscious acts of symbolic communication require a relatively stable social *ground* and a cultural *gravity* governed by codes. Conscious and intentional communication circuits are found in the interior of the brain, as well as out in the open, in the sociocultural spaces that surround humans. Unlike the physical realities of the environment, the sociocultural habitat's ground and gravity have an artificial nature and are much more elastic and unstable than the rigid laws that determine the natural environment. And it is in this artificiality where we may be able to find many of the keys to human consciousness and speech.

And so the following doubt appears: has the brain internalized the properties of the external world? The neurophysiologist Rodolfo Llinás, who considers the brain to be a closed self-referential system modulated by the senses, believes this to be the case. This idea rejects the explanation that the act of walking is a succession of reflexes in a central information input/output system. At the beginning of the twentieth century, Thomas Graham Brown had already demonstrated that organized movement is intrinsically generated without the need for sensory reception and that reflex interaction is only necessary for modulating walking, not for producing it.[12] In 1911 Graham Brown demonstrated that the isolated spinal cord can generate alternate rhythmic impulses in the motor neurons of the hind legs of a cat even in the absence of sensation reception.

---

[11] Edelman, *Bright air, brilliant fire*, pp. 241ff.   [12] Llinás, *I of the vortex*, p. 6.

Today it is believed that there are neuronal networks (central pause generators) capable of generating rhythmic behavior without sensory feedback.[13] Llinás extends this proposal to brain activity in which there would be a neurological apriority that emerged from an internalization process of the external environment that takes the form of an active neuronal wiring. If we transfer this proposal to the question of self-consciousness, we must suppose that – in addition to the properties of the physical world – the human brain has internalized the structures of what I have called social ground and cultural gravity. But it cannot be assumed that there is only one alternative – the internalization proposal as opposed to the reflexology concept, in which learning and cognition of social and cultural elements would be a process of information input and processed answers, a system of data ingestion and order excretion, linking the brain with its environment. There is at least one other interpretation: the proposal that the brain is a system that is open to external cultural circuits and that these circuits are a necessary element for brain function. This situation exists because neuronal spaces are incapable of representing, absorbing, and internalizing the constantly changing properties of culture and of social structure. Only certain components of these properties are part of the neuronal circuits. This does not mean that the brain is a learning machine that goes through life printing information on the blank slate of the mind. Brain evolution was able to adapt to the changing cultural flows (and to certain changes in the physical environment) through the configuration of external circuits closely connected to the internal neuronal structure. It was the gestation of the exocerebrum.

The proposal of a closed self-referential brain that would contain the properties of an external world in an *a priori* manner eliminates the possibility of (and the need for) an exocerebrum to explain the mystery of the self or of consciousness. Subjective experiences and sensations (*qualia*), the same as language, would be intrinsically generated internal brain states. Llinás' proposal discloses the formidable difficulties in describing the brain architecture that underlies the *qualia* and it connects us with the interpretations of Gerald Edelman, Nicholas Humphrey, and Max Velmans that were discussed in chapter 7 and with Ramachandran's imaginary experiment commented on in chapter 6. In order for subjective sensations to be a phenomenon locked up in the brain, it is necessary to demonstrate that the thresholds separating perceptions (of color, weight, tone, etc.) are fixed by internal processes. There is a differential equation from the nineteenth century known as the Weber-Fechner law that appears to establish intensity change perception thresholds of a stimulus: while subjective perceptions increase arithmetically, the objective magnitudes of the

---

[13] Graham Brown, "The intrinsic factors in the act of progression in the mammal." The networks that can generate motor activity rhythmic pause in the absence of sensory information of the peripheral receptors are called CPG (central pattern generators).

corresponding physical stimulus increase geometrically. For example, only a few extra grams are needed in order to notice (while blind-folded) a minimal increase in the weight of a kilogram we are holding. But those same grams are not perceived if we are holding ten kilos: to perceive a change it is necessary to add much more weight. To measure the subjective effects of stimuli, a simple equation can be used that includes a natural logarithm, an experimentally determined constant factor, and the relation between the threshold below which nothing is perceived and the stimulus-induced perceived sensation.[14] A geometric succession of physical sensations for an arithmetic series of subjective thresholds can be determined with this equation, which functions not only with the perception of weight, but also with decibel scales, brightness scales, seven-note tonal series, and other perception scales. Rodolfo Llinás maintains that we can measure *all* the *qualia* or subjective sensations with this equation and thus obtain a mathematical progression that divides experience into subjectively perceived thresholds.[15] He thinks it is applicable to the seven-note musical scale just as – revealing coincidence – to the band of seven colors in the rainbow. Let us stop right there: are there really seven colors in the rainbow? Some dictionaries say so, but actually the thresholds that separate the colors are cultural conventions that vary enormously. Even limiting ourselves to the solar spectrum, and endowed with western eyes, the codes for identifying the chromatic differences will vary, especially in the bands of the bluish section: what color is there between blue and violet? In addition, it will be difficult to find the purple tones that blend at the inner and outer edges of the rainbow. It should be added that the solar spectrum does not include the achromatic colors (black and white) whose symbolism is huge and complex and which happen to be the only colors found in the well-known list of "universal" traits elaborated by the anthropologist Donald E. Brown.[16] Nor does the notion of color appear on this list (in many languages, as in Chinese, there is no word for designating the general category of color).[17] There are languages that have only two basic terms for expressing colors (black and white) and others that have more than ten basic adjectives for designating them. This does not mean that those who speak languages with few words for color have achromatopsia or are backward. Actually, colors for which there are no adjectives can be indicated through the use of nouns or verbs modified by determinant functional morphemes. It is not easy to measure color response in different cultures. There will be an obvious imposition if abstract and artificial chromatic stimuli divided into arbitrary segments and printed on materials foreign to the culture being studied

---

[14] Perception = k · *In* (Ex./Eo), where k is the constant factor, *In* the natural logarithm, Ex is the sensation caused by a stimulus and Eo is the threshold below which no stimulus is perceived.

[15] Llinás, *I of the vortex*, p. 215.   [16] Brown. *Human universals.*

[17] Zahan, "L'homme et la couleur." p. 139.

are used for measuring them. Or when stimuli from elements taken from their customary environment are used, there will be a distortion indirectly provoked by the outside eye that selects and organizes the sample. Despite these difficulties, researchers have been able to discover a wide variety of linguistic encodings for colors that draw upon very varied associations: the color's link with feelings or emotions, the reference to the way in which the thing endowed with color is represented, the impressions it leaves, the peculiarities of the colored object, its relation to another color, to name a very few. In this teeming abundance of symbols and grammatical structures, it is not possible to be guided by equations dealing with the relation between stimuli and sensations: thresholds that separate one chromatic quality from another are not inscribed in the mathematical logic of closed neuronal circuits. The majority of discrete event sequences that are subjectively perceived through sensations cannot be determined through logarithmic stimulus growth, as in the case of the sensation of weight or brightness, but rather through their relation to symbolic networks and syntagmatic chains. Without such relations, it is impossible to understand why the moon is green for certain African ethnic groups, as well as in the poetic universe of the gypsy ballads of Federico García Lorca.

It has been thought that if we strip the brain of subjective devices and cultural supplements, consciousness could be, so to say, at our fingertips. Consciousness would be inside our brain, nestled in brain networks, waiting to be able to express itself. There was a spectacular case in the nineteenth century of a person whose two essential channels of communication with the world were cut off for the first seven years of her life. Helen Keller, born in 1880 in Alabama, became totally blind and deaf at nineteen months of age. At the age of seven she began a tutoring process that seems miraculous and that led her to an extraordinary mastery of the language and culture of her time. In a tender and intelligent book, she describes what she calls "the world I live in." The great psychologist William James, after reading the book, wrote to Helen Keller that he was "quite disconcerted, professionally speaking, by your account of yourself before your 'consciousness' was awakened by instruction," and that he could not understand how she lacked an emotional memory of the period of her life before she began to use the manual alphabet system.[1] Keller herself had written that before the arrival of Anne Sullivan, the teacher who taught her to communicate, she lived "in a world that was a no-world" and she did not think she would ever be able to adequately describe "that unconscious, yet conscious time of nothingness."[2] It seemed that this brilliant woman almost had the memory of her childhood within her reach, the time when she was all but totally devoid of cultural tools that could mark consciousness "in a natural state" with artificial imprints. In a previous book, her fascinating autobiography, Keller points out that, before learning language, she somehow knew that she was different from others. While she used scarcely a dozen rudimentary signs for expressing her wishes, everyone else moved their lips. She states that during this time "the desire to express myself grew."[3] But who was she? Many years later, in a book published in 1955, she dedicated a chapter to correcting her ambiguities. There she practically stops speaking of herself in first person

[1] Letters from December 1908 cited by Roger Shattuck in "A world of words," introduction to Helen Keller's book, *The world I live in* [1908], p. xxviii.
[2] Keller, *The world I live in*, p. 72.   [3] Keller, *The story of my life* [1903], p. 22.

and states that before language she was a "no-person" and she refers to this being by the name of Phantom. However, she has some recollection of that phantasmal being and even comes to write paradoxically that there are images in her memory of the place where her teacher began to show her how to use manual alphabet signs: "I am conscious of a Phantom lost in what seemed to her new surroundings."[4] Little Helen had certain autistic traits that unquestionably came from the absence of important social ties. Her teacher relates, for example, that she "refused to be caressed and there was no way of appealing to her affection or sympathy or childish love of approbation."[5]

Upon reading the unsettling pages in which Helen Keller describes her prelinguistic condition, we feel that her consciousness, just when we thought we were on the verge of understanding it in its primeval state, slips through our fingers like a phantasmal fluid unable to be grasped. But soon we understand that we are reading the testimony of a woman who used her hands – in substitution of the senses she lacked – to build her own consciousness. Keller's fascinating experience is how, through a single channel (touch) and at a spectacular speed, she went a distance that normal children using all their senses take longer to accomplish. This is why, in the famous passage of the well, her story is so fascinating from the instant she understands for the first time the relation between symbols and things. The water that was pumped from the well did not escape through Helen's fingers: at that mythic moment she understood that the combination of signs that her teacher spelled out in her one hand symbolized the cool liquid that was pouring out over the other. There she forever held onto the fluid that connected her to the world. That night, for the first time, she gave her teacher a kiss. Helen Keller's story makes it clearer to see how consciousness is constructed as a prosthesis revolving around the axis of language. This prosthesis, that substituted hearing and sight, was first the very old manual alphabet system of signs that the Trappist monks had invented in order to communicate with each other despite their vow of silence and that later was adapted for teaching the deaf. The system had already been used with a certain amount of success on a woman in Boston, Laura Bridgeman, who became blind and deaf at a very early age and who was made famous by Charles Dickens in a memorable story of his visit to the United States in 1842. Then afterwards, the Braille alphabet enormously expanded Keller's conscious world and enabled her to become a remarkable writer.

Helen Keller's experience is an example, full of rich and spirited nuances, of the hypothesis with which I began my reflections. I have described an imaginary brain in "a natural state" confronted by problems that exceed its capacity. Such a

---

[4] Keller, *Teacher* [1955], chapter 2, reproduced in *The story of my life*, p. 397.
[5] "Anne Sullivan's letters and reports," letter dated March 11, 1887, in Keller, *The story of my life*, p. 143.

brain undergoes considerable suffering, like that of the Keller child who became furious and cried when she encountered difficulties. A brain under these conditions, left only to its inner forces, turns off. This is what happened to another girl, Genie, who in 1970 showed up with her mother at a social work office in Los Angeles. The child was 13 years old and her father had kept her, from the age of 20 months, locked in a room, tied down in a straitjacket, isolated from the family that he did not allow to speak to her, and beaten if she made a sound. Genie was neither blind nor deaf but she had not been able to have any type of social relation with her environment. When released from her prison, she could understand only a few dozen words and hardly spoke, she was unable to chew food, she weighed only 27 kilograms, was 137 centimeters tall and could not fix her gaze further than 3.5 meters, she was incontinent and, apparently, she could not even cry.[6] For several years Genie was treated and observed by various psychiatrists, psychologists, and linguists. She was transferred from the hospital to a home where she received maternal care and she began to learn some words, though after five years she reached a limit in her verbal skills that she was never able to surpass. Although she never mastered syntax (she could barely construct a few phrases with verbs and nouns), she developed a sharp visual intelligence and certain mathematical abilities. But after five years she was incapable of assimilating the pronominal system. She used "I" and "you" indistinctly and arbitrarily interchanged different pronouns.[7] Her capacity to understand social norms was minimal; for example, Genie frequently masturbated in public, something which made everyone extremely uncomfortable. Due to her mental limitations and the instability brought on by the frequent changing of adoptive homes, as the years went by this girl gradually fell into a gloomy silence. She ended up being transferred to an institution for disabled adults in southern California where she lives submerged in depression, removed from the world. Her brain motor, unable to overcome the challenges, turned off.

Why did Genie not manage to develop as Helen Keller was able to? The most accepted explanation, apart from the incredible abuse and neglect the child endured, alludes to the fact that the critical period for learning a language ends at puberty. Therefore Genie was no longer able to build the exocerebral connections necessary for developing advanced semantic and syntactic abilities. Neurological tests showed that Genie's scant use of language was sustained in the right brain hemisphere and that large areas of the left side appeared to be shut off.[8] Perhaps the Neanderthals were like her: intelligent beings but lacking neuronal circuits dependent on the sociocultural environment that are capable of stimulating exocerebral connections. The case of Genie would seem to show that there are no inborn grammatical structures printed in some brain module

[6] See Russ Rymer's book *Genie*.   [7] Curtiss, *Genie*.
[8] Leiber, "Nature's experiments, society's closures."

and that syntax, as well as meanings, is built in a network connecting neuronal circuits with cultural networks.[9] This does not mean that the brain is a blank slate. Circuits that need to be connected to the external environment without a doubt have genetically determined characteristics and stable signaling systems.

Let us now look, with very different examples, at the way in which the use of cultural prostheses helps dramatic pathological situations to be managed. This happens in patients with Parkinson's disease and those who have had encephalitis who use what A. R. Luria called "behavior algorithms" and what Oliver Sacks defines as conduct prostheses – artificial substitutes based on calculations – to keep from becoming "frozen" along the way as they move around.[10] The patients calculate paths in a space that let them throw themselves about a room as if they were billiard balls in such a way that when they bounce off the walls they end up in the spot where they wanted to be. Sacks adds that music works as a better prosthesis (a peculiar pacemaker) than these algorithms and, for example, impels patients to recover what Luria called the "cynetic melody" of normal writing, when without music they were not able to make more than illegible lines.[11]

These examples show us once again the key position of speech and language in the exocerebral circuits. Symbolic communication systems become the nucleus around which pieces of the exocerebrum are articulated. Some linguists consider it to be a hard nucleus, essentially made up of formal syntactic structures that originate, as Chomsky has assured, in a genetic device installed in the mind, dedicated to language acquisition and learning. From this perspective, a brain with no specialized inborn module would not suffice for a child to be able to acquire a complex grammatical system in a very short time from the few expressions and words that it hears in the family environment (this argument is the so-called "poverty of the stimulus"). This reasoning has been generalized to include a large variety of abilities and cultural traits, making it seemingly necessary for there to be modules for friendship and for child-care, as well as for fear and social exchange.[12] The modular theory can be sustained only by accepting the supposition that essential language structures fit completely inside the brain (and by extension, that practically all the bases of the cultural world are also housed within the cranium). I sustain, in contrast, that linguistic structures function as a mediating nucleus in the exocerebral circuits. Many neurologists have found it incredibly difficult to integrate the formalist,

[9] Of course there are linguists who do not agree that Genie's language was ungrammatical and syntactically defective and inconsistent since this goes against Chomskyan postulates. See Jones, "Contradictions and unanswered questions in the Genie case."

[10] Luria, *The man with a shattered world*, last chapter. Sacks, *Awakenings*, p. 229n. See also Thaut, *Rhythm, music, and the brain*.

[11] Sacks, *Awakenings.*, p. 280.

[12] Tooby and Cosmides, "The psychological foundations of culture."

rigid, and hard vision of language centered on its grammatical expression into their research. I believe that neurology will find a much more stimulating and creative inspiration in reflections based on the symbolism of speech. In the mathematical logic tradition of Alfred North Whitehead, the philosopher Susanne Langer has proposed a brilliant interpretation of speech and the so-called artistic and mythological languages.[13] I wish to retrieve her idea that language is the discursive part of a set of symbolic expressions such as rituals, dance, music, the fine arts, and myth. A similar idea can be retaken from Ernst Cassirer.[14] Langer proposes that a general theory of symbolism should make a distinction between two symbolic modes: the discursive and the non-discursive, the verbal and non-verbal. The two modes come from the same root, Langer maintains, but their flowers are different: "in this physical, space-time world of our experience there are things which do not fit the grammatical scheme of expression. But they are not necessarily blind, inconceivable, mystical affairs; they are simply matters which require to be conceived through some symbolistic schema other than discursive language."[15] She goes so far as to say that "if ritual is the cradle of language, metaphor is the law of its life." Language must have emerged and evolved in a symbolic context of rituals, dances, festivities, and music, in other words, in an environment of non-discursive expressions.[16]

Accordingly, it is important to distinguish between signs and symbols. To make the distinction Langer cites precisely the famous passage in Helen Keller's autobiography where she relates the discovery of the difference between signals or digital signs and the name or symbol of the thing (water). The sign or signal, which is the basis of animal intelligence, indicates something about what has to be acted upon, or it is a means by which to stimulate an action. In contrast the symbol is an instrument of thought.[17] A signal reveals the presence of a thing, a situation, an event, or a condition. The signal is perceived

---

[13] Langer, *Philosophy in a new key*. This book, now almost forgotten, was extraordinarily successful when it appeared in 1942 and is a good text aimed at the educated layperson. Guillermo Lorenzo has pointed out the importance of Langer's ideas about the origin of language: "El origen del lenguaje como sobresalto natural."

[14] Cassirer, *Myth and language* [1924].   [15] Langer, *Philosophy in a new key*, p. 88.

[16] *Ibid.*, p. 141. Steven Mithen has stressed the role of music in the origin of language, although without paying much attention to Langer's ideas. Mithen offers a very speculative modular interpretation and an attractive examination of recent neurophysiological studies about music and its possible relation to hominid evolution (*The singing Neanderthals*). In a previous book *The prehistory of the mind*, he had offered an overview of the possible origin of the human mind, but he had not realized the importance of symbolic non-discursive expressions such as music.

[17] Langer does not use the concept of sign in the same way as Saussure, who conceived of it as the union between an acoustic image and a concept, between a sensory representation and an abstract idea. Sign for Saussure is a dual entity that connects the signifiers (patterns of sound) with the signified (concepts). For Langer this is symbolic function and the sign is more like the symptom or the signal. To avoid confusion I will preferably use the concept of signal. Langer, *Philosophy in a new key*, p. 63.

by the subject and signifies a present, future, or past object. A certain smell indicates the presence of a fruit, a distinct noise means that a large quadruped is approaching, a peculiar taste reveals that a food is spoiled. In addition to these natural signals there are artificial signs: the whistle announcing the departure of a train, the two letters signifying a syllabic vowel sound, the points on a stave signifying a precise musical chord. Helen Keller learned various sequences of digital signs before understanding that they formed a symbol (a word) that she could use to think and conceive an object. As Langer sustains, signs *announce* their objects to a subject, while symbols *lead to their being conceived*. A short sequence of signals in the hand could announce to Keller that a cold sensation would flow through her fingers, but only the word "water" as a symbol enabled her to think it. The most obvious and simple symbols are proper names that evoke a concrete person. Of course, signals can be used as symbols, and symbols can function as signals or signs. But it is important to recognize the difference between symbolic functions and signaling functions.

The difference between signals and symbols is important when confronting the problem of the connections between the brain and the exocerebrum. Neuronal circuits function by means of chemical and electrical signals, while language is a symbolic system. As far as is currently known, the brain does not function through symbols, at least not directly, or through representation processes: in order to operate through symbols the nervous system needs to be connected with the cultural environment so that certain signal conglomerates adopt a symbolic form. But it is not yet known how this transformation works. As for cultural systems, operations with signals that are transformed into symbolic representations do take place within them. My proposal suggests that some symbolic transformations of cultural circuits have a *cerebral character*, so to speak, without their being operations that take place inside the cranium. They occur in the networks that connect brains with one another, individuals with one another.

In order to understand this aspect of the problem it may be useful to move away from the more rigid facets of encoded language and approach fluent and flexible expressions of speech. It has been correctly observed that the great capacity children have for learning a language (which supposedly proves that there is a brain module that generates linguistic structures) refers to spontaneous forms of everyday speech. But when generative analysis is applied to syntax, examples of written and encoded language are always used. The problem is that there is a very big difference between spontaneous speech and encoded language.[18] So there really is no abyss between the "poverty" of linguistic context that stimulates the child and the "wealth" of syntactic rules of everyday speech.

---

[18] Li and Hombert, "On the evolutionary origin of language," p. 198.

It is completely possible in the socialization process to gradually move up from common and simple speech to the management of sophisticated linguistic structures without the need for a specialized brain module guiding the operations of learning.[19]

Let us now take a look at another interpretation that complements the analysis: that of Lev Vygotsky, who published a pioneer text entitled *Thought and speech* in 1934.[20] Vygotsky does not conceive the development of thought as the gradual socialization of profoundly intimate and personal states (as posited by Piaget). For Vygotsky the primordial function of speech, in children as well as in adults, lies in communication and social contact. Early forms of speech are essentially social; during growth, the child continually transfers these originally social behavior patterns to its internal processes.[21] The development of spoken language begins as a social activity, later it acquires a self-centered character in order to finally generate inner speech. For Vygotsky it is important to recognize that the grammars of normal speech, of written language, and of inner speech are very different. Colloquial speech uses very simple syntax, has an expressive and musical character full of intonations and implicit suppositions, and is always developed as part of a fluent conversation motivated by speakers and the context in which it is produced. In contrast, inner speech has a condensed, abbreviated, and almost totally predicative character, given that the thinking subject is always known by the thinker and does not need to be expressed in precise form.[22] Inner speech has an incomplete and disconnected syntax. Written and encoded language, however, has a very complex and coherent syntax with a strong monological and abstract inclination. From Vygotsky we can understand that linguistic structures are diverse and flexible, they are not expressed in just one way, they adapt to different functions, and they are situated at different planes of complexity.

Human symbolic expressions are not limited to language and speech. The plastic abilities that enable drawing, painting, sculpting, and engraving have generated a wide variety of symbols. The same is true for music and dance. In these non-discursive forms of expression we find a relation between significant signals and symbols, but we do not find, as in language, the minimum units of meaning (words) that can be combined in sequences that have their equivalent in different languages. Colors, images, body movements, or tones are not part of

---

[19] The difference between *language* and *speech* is similar but not identical to Saussure's distinction between *langue* (abstract system) and *parole* (system manifestation). The difference that I am interested in emphasizes planes of complexity and functions.

[20] The 1986 English edition has kept the erroneous title *Thought and language* due to the fact that it was widely known by this title from the first translation from 1962 (I cite the 1986 version revised by Alex Kozulin). Also see the book *Language and cognition* by A. R. Luria, Vygotsky's great continuer.

[21] Lev Vygotsky, *Thought and language*, pp. 34–35.   [22] *Ibid.*, p. 182.

vocabulary, and the structures that join them are not syntax. And nevertheless these expressions form symbolic flows or conglomerates that evoke feelings, ideas, and emotions by non-representative means. If we wish to understand symbolic expressions as components of the exocerebrum, we must not think only of their complex and sophisticated forms that are characteristics of advanced civilizations. We do not need to analyze the art of, let us say, Dmitri Shostakovich, Isadora Duncan, and Pablo Picasso as part of the exocerebrum. However, we must accept the fact that at least part, perhaps a small part, of modern symbolic expressions (both discursive and non-discursive) is closely linked to neuronal networks that rely on the existence of external connections. This small part of the exocerebral symbolism is that which we can suppose was already present when the first humans began to make statuettes, paint cave walls, and probably to sing, dance, and speak. How does a neuroscientist approach the world of art? Dr. Ramachandran dedicates an entertaining chapter of his book on consciousness to art and I am interested in citing it, because an important part of his reflection is inspired by animal behavior when confronted by a prosthesis. He takes the example from Nikolaas Tinbergen, who carried out some experiments on herring gull chicks. Just barely out of their shells they begin to peck at the red spot on their mother's yellow beak; she then regurgitates semi-digested food to feed her young. The chick obviously reacts in this way due to the fact that certain nervous circuits in the visual zone of its brain are specialized in recognizing gull beaks. In the course of his experiments, Tinbergen presented an artificial beak with a red spot to the chicks and they reacted in exactly the same manner, even when the scientist's hand, instead of their mother, was behind the beak. But Tinbergen took things to the extreme: he took a large yellow stick with three red stripes and showed it to the chicks. They reacted with still greater enthusiasm in front of this curious artifact that did not even look like a gull beak: they preferred the prosthesis to the real beak. And this is where Ramachandran's idea comes in: "If herring-gulls had an art gallery, they would hang a large stick with three red stripes on the wall; they would worship it, pay millions of dollars for it, they would call it a Picasso, but would not understand why they are mesmerized by this thing even though it doesn't resemble anything."[23] An ethnologist studying Ramachandran's speculations could ask himself: why does this neurologist think that art lovers who buy contemporary art act just like gull chicks? Because he is convinced that there is a perceptual grammar that contains universal primitive figural elements, one of which is the attraction for representations in which certain significant features have been hyper-emphasized to the point of being completely deformed (like the yellow stick with three red stripes). The extended attraction among many

---

[23] Ramachandran, *A brief tour of human consciousness*, p. 47.

neurologists to the idea of mental modules that function as archetypes, and that interest them more than the prostheses and artifacts that they eventually rely on, is very symptomatic. This attraction is justified by the evidence that there are a good number of symbolic operations that have their basis in neuronal circuits. Ramachandran considers there to be various signs that "sensory metaphors" are inserted in the nervous system, as demonstrated by synesthetic phenomena that connect areas of the brain that are usually separate (I have already commented on the association between numbers and colors).[24] He mentions three tests. First, the links between sounds and images that seem to be deeply rooted in the brain, such as the one established between the sounds *booba* and *kiki*: 98 percent of people (from different cultures) associate these two sounds with a bulbous figure similar to an amoeba and a jagged figure with an uneven and shattered edge, respectively. This and other examples would demonstrate that we are facing the previous existence of a non-arbitrary translation of the visual appearance of an object (represented in the fusiform gyrus) and the representation of a sound (in the auditory cortex).[25] Second, he supposes an association between the visual area and Broca's area (that controls vocalization muscles); for example, a test would be that the small objects are symbolized in different languages with words that make the lips imitate the sound ("diminutive") and big things that force the mouth to open ("enormous," "large"). To this not very convincing argument he adds a third association between the areas of the hand and the mouth, which are known to be adjacent in the homunculus motor drawn by Penfield. Darwin had already observed that people frequently move their jaws unconsciously when cutting with scissors.

An essential aspect needs to be considered in these examples, including the case of the chick that accepts a stick as a metaphor of the maternal gull bringing it food: the presence of an external symbolic artificial element, a prosthesis that appears in the form of a drawing, a word, an instrument, or a simulation (of a beak). I have no doubt that the use of these prostheses relies on processes of synesthesia in the brain. This internal synesthetic process operates through electrical and chemical signals that travel between regions (motor regions of speech, visual centers, and the fusiform gyrus). But in my opinion it is very difficult to suppose that correspondence relationships between regions utilize symbolic and metaphoric codes. The internal flow of signals needs to be able to establish synesthetic connections with external symbolic prostheses, as opposed to doing so only between different areas of the brain.

Let us go back to the mental experiment of gulls interested in art. For them to have gotten to the point of forming a society willing to organize exhibits, they

---

[24] *Ibid.*, p. 62.   [25] *Ibid.*, p. 77.

had to fabricate symbolic prostheses themselves that enable them to have a stable cawing system for communicating with each other, in addition to many other devices and social institutions. Perhaps a mutant group of gulls understood the importance of Tinbergen's simulation and was gradually able to develop into an advanced civilization from that divine breath of sorts. But the first evolutionary steps of a hypothetical group of intelligent social gulls would have to be the development of a minimal package of exocerebral prostheses to be able to survive in a dangerous environment. To this end the cultured gulls (just like primitive humans) would have to have some kind of system enabling them to link and establish connections between internal signals and external symbols. Gull or human self-awareness would appear when this step from inner signals to external symbols that are understood by other individuals was produced.

When Ramachandran approaches this problem he proposes an idea that, had he examined it thoroughly, would have led him directly to the exocerebrum. He suggests that unconscious sensory representations acquire the condition of *qualia* during the process of being encoded into manageable sets that can reach the central executive structures of the brain. This produces other high-level representations that he calls "meta-representations" and that can be considered "almost as a second 'parasitic' brain" that allows for more economic descriptions of the automatic processes that the first brain carries out.[26] There are two alternatives here: to propose a kind of internal and private homunculus, or to go a step further and imagine that this second brain is external. Ramachandran accepts the first option and believes that the cerebral homunculus is responsible for carrying out representations of representations (that is: metarepresentations) and therefore is tied to linguistic abilities. It seems necessary for consciousness to come into being in a type of jump from one kind of representation to another. But some neurologists, like Ramachandran, are afraid that the jump will catapult them into external space, outside of the nervous circuits. They prefer to remain inside the brain even when that means having to embrace the Cartesian homunculus in its metarepresentational incarnation as a translating and mediating structure.[27]

The need to turn to the hypothesis of a second internal brain that would have emerged during the course of evolution is to me symptomatic and revealing. Without a doubt at some point of the evolutionary process new circuits arose

---

[26] *Ibid.*, p. 99.

[27] Ramachandran admits that even though the "I" is private it is greatly enriched through social interaction and he accepts the fact that it is possible for it to have evolved principally in a social environment. Furthermore, he believes our brains are inextricably tied to the cultural atmosphere. But society and culture are vaguely defined as "environment" or "atmosphere" without recognizing that there are structures and circuits in this habitat that can form part of that 'parasitic' brain. *Ibid.*, pp. 105 and 108.

and the previous ones adapted to high-level cognitive operations, but the strictly metarepresentational functions require sociocultural external sources. What we are looking for are symbols that represent signals, and signals capable of indicating the presence of symbols. In order to do this, let us return to the problem of visual images that enable certain facets of art to be understood. We can understand that the brain's attraction to certain exaggerated and deformed features (the gulls' yellow stick with the three stripes) is expressed in humans, for example, in anthropomorphic figures with enlarged sexual features such as the famous prehistoric Venuses or phallic representations. Here, there would be a connection between a certain signal selectivity with which nervous circuits work and symbols tied to the fertility cult. Neuronal preference for certain chromatic associations can be tied to tribal or familial identity. The inclination and ability to discover figures in camouflaged contexts (a predator hidden in the foliage) can be connected to symbols of concealed evil powers. The ability to appreciate isolated elements out of context can be associated with symbolic capacities to create names and nouns. For the esthete gulls, the oft-cited stick with stripes that grabs the attention of their neurons is a symbol of the primordial mother. In order for these particular transformations to take place, the sequences of neuronal signals need to be expressed as symbols that are understood by other individuals; and vice versa: symbolic structures coming out of society must be able to find an equivalent in signals capable of circulating through the nervous system. I am inclined to think that the "translating apparatus" is found outside the cranium for one simple reason: as far as we know the brain is only capable of processing signals, while we can be sure that social and cultural circuits can operate as symbols and as signals. Of course a discrete sequence of neuronal signals, equivalent to a symbol, must be accompanied by some kind of "marker" that identifies it, so that its meaning is not diluted by the torrent of electrical and chemical codes. I will tackle this problem later on when I refer to the subject of memory.

10   Outside and inside: the immense blue

In order to understand the relationship between exocerebral networks and neuronal circuits that operate through electrical and chemical signals, apparently it is necessary to find certain devices that connect the internal and external sequences. The first difficulty we run into is in the separation itself of the internal and the external. Two important interpretations of mental processes have been developed, but each one emphasizes the opposite sphere. First of all, we have the so-called "internalist" view that states that consciousness is a process determined by certain types of internal brain activity in individuals during the process of their interaction with the world. In contrast, the "externalist" view says that consciousness is a construct that depends on language-based social and cultural relations. The first view tends to be innatist and maintains that cognitive structures are genetically determined brain devices. It is the view held by Noam Chomsky and Jerry Fodor.[1] At the other extreme we find authors such as Clifford Geertz and Richard Lewontin who emphasize the decisive importance of interaction and the symbolic system.[2] I do not wish to examine this polemic because, among other reasons, it seems to me to be a confrontation that has long been surpassed, much like the opposition between nature and culture.

But not all neuroscientists, deep down, are convinced that the nature/culture opposition has been overcome, because that means accepting that the mind and consciousness go beyond the cranial and epidermal borders defining the individual. And for many, accepting that would be the equivalent of validating the "externalist" view. Recently Robert Wilson, known for his reflections on the cognitive sciences, has dedicated an interesting book to the problem of the boundaries of the mind. Wilson is convinced that the mind does not come to a stop in front of the walls that separate the individual from the external world,

---

[1] See Chomsky, *New horizons in the study of language and mind*, and Fodor, *The modularity of mind*.

[2] See Geertz, *The interpretation of cultures*, and Lewontin, *Biology as ideology*. In another essay Geertz referred to the "functionally incomplete character of the nervous system" ("Culture, mind, brain / Brain, mind, culture," p. 205). An especially interesting and creative approach can be found in Clark, *Supersizing the mind*.

and presents a hypothesis that coincides to a certain degree with the ideas I have expressed about the exocerebrum.[3] Wilson conceives of consciousness as a process extended in time (lasting much longer than a few seconds) that is supported by an external environmental and cultural *scaffolding*. According to Wilson this process is *embodied* in a physical body that is *embedded* in an environment. Unfortunately he does not elaborate on the explanation of the external scaffolding that forms a part of consciousness. He cites navigation equipment, watches, and maps, and of course speech and writing, as examples of mediators that modify the structure of cognition.[4] The conception that consciousness is supported by cultural and environmental scaffolding is similar to my idea that human self-consciousness operates through cultural prostheses. But the idea that the prostheses (or scaffolding) constitute a symbolic substitution system that the brain circuits cannot complete on their own is missing from Wilson's assessment.

Let us now look at the problem from the perspective of computational models of consciousness. Wilson reflects on the broad view that not only considers the brain to be a computational system but also believes that said system includes the environment surrounding the organism. The problem with this interpretation is that in order for it to be coherent, the mind, as well as the world that surrounds it, must be thought of as a unified computational system. But for that to be true, there is a requisite: the social environment and neuronal circuits must constitute a complex causal structure that enables there to be a common formal characterization in such a way that it is unnecessary to look for translation rules between parts of the brain and environmental expressions.[5] Even though the computational model of the mind and the brain has been abandoned by almost all neurobiologists, the question of a possible systemic unit of internal and external spheres of consciousness continues to be a disquieting theme. Regarding this, Dana Ballard's explanation of the functions of rapid and constant updating of data that are encoded in the environment during the cognition process is attractive. The brain takes advantage of information that is stored in the environment and therefore does not need to be filed or computed by the individual. An example of this "deictic encoding" in the visual recognition process are the rapid and constant eye movements, saccadic movements that obtain information from looking directly at certain fixed points of a contour – information that does not need to be kept inside the brain. Thus the optic environmental order is taken advantage of by rapid eye movements that directly point to or signal the elements of the visual field that are needed to complete a process of cognition

---

[3] Wilson, *Boundaries of the mind*.
[4] Wilson calls his concept of consciousness TESEE: temporally extended, scaffolded, and embodied and embedded.
[5] Wilson, *Boundaries of the mind*, pp. 167–169.

and recognition.[6] This interpretation can be extended to memory, attention, and other activities.

A difficult obstacle to overcome is the fact that codes require a syntax that organizes the way in which they should be combined and managed. As Wilson observes, codes need to be interpreted and therefore require other codes to carry out the deciphering. But here, we enter into an infinite regression, since new codes will always be needed to decipher the ones before them. Or to overcome this obstacle we can imagine a non-interpretative process that gets by without codes: but in this case the use of codes in the interaction does not serve any purpose, since no subsequent process will try to decipher and interpret them.[7] If we take this last alternative to an extreme, we could arrive at a dead-end: social and cultural coding would be a strange external epiphenomenon that would not have an influence on the functioning of neuronal circuits which would operate through non-interpretive and non-representational internal processes. But that does not solve the problem of the links between the internal and external. It simply annuls it by declaring a categorical divorce between two immanent spheres: the external cultural environment and the cerebral space.

In my opinion, the problem scientific research should resolve consists of finding the specific way in which nervous circuits – and specifically the cerebral cortex – are able to work with the symbols, codes, and signals of the cultural world. There have been great advances in research in locating the processes initiated in the sensory stimuli that are transduced in the peripheral terminals of nerve fibers and sent to primary sensory areas of the cerebral cortex. As Mountcastle explains, the geography and the connections of nerve impulses are relatively well known, but very little is known about the operative mechanisms and processes. Many phenomena have been localized in the cerebral cortex, such as synchronization, data accumulation and recovery, amplification, and others. But the neuronal circuits of these processes are not yet completely understood. The fact is, the basic functions of the cerebral cortex are not known.[8] Mountcastle points out the urgent need to create theoretical models and hypotheses that guide research and he underlines the effectiveness of computational models in stimulating neurophysiological studies. However, he categorically asserts that the metaphor that sees the brain as a digital computer is totally false and should be abandoned.[9]

I believe that new reflections by scientists on the questions of consciousness contribute to the conception and development of stimulating and creative

---

[6] Ballard, Hayhoe, Pook and Rao, "Deictic codes for the embodiment of cognition." See Robert Wilson's commentaries in *Boundaries of the Mind*, pp. 176ff.
[7] Wilson, *Boundaries of the Mind*, pp. 140–149.
[8] Mountcastle, "Brain science at the century's ebb," pp. 16–17.   [9] *Ibid.*, p. 29.

theoretical models. Something I would like to emphasize is the fact that high-level consciousness (or self-consciousness) seems to contain a paradox: in order for individuals to be aware of their unique individuality, their "internal" sensations must be exposed to the "external" world. I am not referring to the obvious fact that the brain nourishes itself with information that comes from the environment. Rather, I mean that the unitary nature of the internal information flow is confirmed to the degree in which it comes into contact with and circulates through the social and cultural space, interacting with other people. An organism's individuality is not solely defined by the epidermis. In other words: in order for an individuality to be able to define its internal world, it is also necessary for this world to be external and exposed to the inclemency of the social climate. But if the interior is also outside, at least partially, then the internal-external dichotomy begins to lose meaning. I have already pointed out that Paul Ricoeur, in his discussion with Jean-Pierre Changeux, suggested that consciousness is outside of itself, and that it is necessary to recognize that conscious space is not found in its entirety within the brain. Changeux defends the usefulness of consciousness models that define it as processes that occur within the cranium. Ricoeur points out to him that the model he postulates does not come from the neurosciences, but rather from other disciplines that precisely stress the point of an opening to a world formed by interactions, and that allows consciousness to be seen as a space of simulation and virtual actions that is interspersed between the external world and the organism. And nevertheless, Changeux, like many other neuroscientists, is paradoxically convinced that "all of that takes place inside the brain."[10] Ricoeur reminds him that the space of consciousness is tied to time and therefore to live human experience, whose vital space is on the one hand that of people's bodies, their postures, their movements, and their moving about; but on the other hand, is also the surrounding external space. This global space of live experience is private and common, corporeal and public. For Ricoeur the so-called "internal cerebral environment" is found within that wide space that includes the organism, as well as its inhabitable environment.[11]

An attempt has been made to overcome the paradox of consciousness through metapsychological theorizations that define the "I" as the development in the child of a figurative representation of itself from the experience of the surface of the skin. That is the definition of the "Skin-Ego" made by the psychoanalyst Didier Anzieu, who, afraid of seeing psychology become neurophysiology's poor relation, attempts to place consciousness of the "I" in the skin – an originary fact from both a biological and imaginary viewpoint. For Anzieu the Skin-Ego is a phantasmal reality, an intermediary structure between

---

[10] Changeux and Ricoeur, *Ce qui nous fait penser*, pp. 155 and 157.   [11] *Ibid.*, p. 158.

the body, psychism, the world, and the others.[12] The skin as a metaphor for the form of the ego can be stimulating, but it does not cease to be a false solution to the consciousness paradox. It is only a curious wordplay, where the skin is a covering, such as the peel of a fruit or the cerebral cortex, full of folds and invaginations, that holds the individual organism within its limits. The ego would be housed in a psychic skin endowed with the structure of a cover, a notion that would enable psychoanalysts to better diagnose the illnesses of their present-day patients who suffer less from neuroses, phobias, and hysterias and more from narcissistic anguishes characteristic of people who do not recognize the limits and boundaries separating the psychic "I" from the corporeal, the ideal "I" from reality, or that which depends on oneself from that which depends on others.[13] But the fact that modern and postmodern culture appears to make people more vulnerable to narcissistic wounds supposedly caused by defects and weaknesses of the psychic covering does not shed any light on the question of consciousness: instead it helps us define certain peculiarities of the complex transition toward a new cultural and sociopolitical culture whose codes, at the beginning of the twenty-first century, we do not yet know.

Metaphors are useful for stimulating research and reflection. I believe the problem of the internal-external dichotomy in the cognitive process and in the formation of self-consciousness can be thought about more thoroughly with the metaphor of the Klein bottle that I have mentioned before. A Klein bottle – named in honor of the great German mathematician – is the result of an action similar to that carried out on a flat strip of paper to create the Möbius band, where the back and front are the same side. If both ends of the strip that has been twisted once are joined together, that unsettling three-dimensional geometric space that has only one side is formed. The so-called Klein bottle is a topological space obtained by joining the two ends of a tube, bending it in such a way that it does not form a ring and therefore has only one side. In a space of this kind we can move from one side to the other without having to go across the surface: it is a bottle where one moves from the inside to the outside without ever having to go out.

Many neuroscientists reject this paradoxical situation. For example, for Antonio Damasio the mind and its consciousness are first and foremost private phenomena, even though they offer many public signs of their existence. Therefore he tells us: "I will never know your thoughts, unless you tell me, and you will never know mine until I tell you."[14] But things are not so simple: my answer to him would be "if you do not explain it to anyone, you will not know *that* you think, even though you know *what* you think." But since we humans are not isolated creatures, but rather talking individuals who do not stop communicating with one another, we know *what* we think and we realize *that* we think. Therefore

[12] Anzieu, *Le moi-peau*, pp. 25–26.   [13] *Ibid.*, p. 29.
[14] Damasio, *The feeling of what happens*, p. 309.

the well-known mental experiment of the scientist who is an expert in the neuro-physiology of color but shuts herself up in a black and white atmosphere is of no use to us. Supposedly one day this expert goes out to another world and experiences the sensation of color for the first time. The conclusion is that her scientific knowledge, no matter how refined, cannot give her the unique and exclusively private multi-chromatic experience.[15] Therefore it is supposed that color consciousness is internal and not able to be transferred. Ramachandran's solution to this problem was discussed in chapter 5. Now, the only thing this mental experiment tells us is that it is not possible for chromatic experiences to be communicated through a detailed description of neuronal circuits and their scientific explanation. But if we escape from the mental laboratory where the experiment is artificially carried out and we approach the cultural networks, we can prove that human beings communicate chromatic experience (and many other kinds) with one another on a daily basis.

Social coexistence surrounds us with enormous swarms of color-related symbols. Fragments of songs, phrases, memories of paintings, or movies, verses, dresses, jewels, and a thousand other things are connected to our notion of, for example, blue. One could say that there is a small segment of the exocerebrum applied to blue and a writer can take advantage of this to write a story or poem that transmits his experience of color, through analogies, metaphors, implicit codes, presuppositions, and suppositions. When we read Rubén Darío's book *Blue*, the poet transmits to us, among many other things, his sensations about blue. Of course, he does not transmit his *entire* experience of blue, only a portion, a fragment that propels a flow of the poet's own ideas and emotions that we do not know before reading his work. In his mental experiment, Ramachandran would plug an artificial nerve cable directly connected to our neuronal system, into Rubén Darío's brain: in this way we would have the *entire* poetic experience of blue felt by this writer, who would have been converted into a mechanical and automatic prosthesis. In this imaginary example we would obtain the blue experience of an individual born in Nicaragua in the nineteenth century, but we would lose the modernist sensations of his symbolistic text:

> Oh immense blue! I worship
> your gleeful cloudage
> and the subtle gold dust mist
> where fragrances and dreams end.   ("Anagke," 1888)[16]

Where is consciousness here? It is precisely in the indirect symbolic connection between Rubén Darío's impressions and our experience when reading his

---

[15] See Jackson, "Epiphenomenal qualia," and the commentaries of Antonio Damasio, *The feeling of what happens*, p. 307.
[16] English translation done specially for this book by the poet Sam Abrams.

verses. It is the same incomplete and fragmentary character of communication that allows me to say that the subtle mist, gleeful cloudage, and fragrances and dreams are blue-related symbols that form part of the subjective consciousness and therefore are not locked up in the brains of the man who wrote them and of those who read them. They are also found in the books and libraries of the great cultural memory of a society. Thus, we can partially have access to the mental processes of Rubén Darío and other people. And I stress that we only have partial access: if access to the consciousness of others were total, paradoxically we would lose our sense of identity and our consciousness would erode.

Let us move on now to a small simulation of neurophysiological interpretation. If we read these verses to a monolingual Japanese speaker, only the primary and secondary auditory areas of that person's brain would be activated. In the next phase of the experiment we read a disjointed list of nouns, adjectives, and verbs taken from the poem to an English speaker:

fragrances	blue	gold
mist	dust	immense
gleeful	dreams	worship

In this case there is comprehensible lexical-semantic information and the consequent brain reaction is more extensive: the left inferior frontal circumvolution is activated, among other zones. The next step is to read the following strange, abnormal, and difficult to understand verses to the same person:

Oh worfosh argal! I subship
your stedful clidoge
and the abtle cheld fust oost

In this case the effort to decipher the sense of some unknown words, but inserted in phrases with comprehensible grammatical information, activates the two temporal poles, in addition to the auditory areas, and a much greater activity in the left hemisphere is observed. Another pattern of brain activity would appear if the semantic information were correct, but the syntactic structure were mutilated:

I worships those dusting gleeful
why fragrant immense and ended

Finally, we read the poem to our subject just as Darío wrote it: extensive and important activity appears in many regions of the brain, especially in the left prefrontal area.[17]

---

[17] The mental experiment is a paraphrase of actual scientific studies. See Neville and Bavelier, "Specificity and plasticity in neurocognitive development in humans," and Changeux, *L'homme de vérité*, p. 190.

All of this indicates that our brain responds in an orderly fashion and that there are behavior patterns that are recognized in the topographic distribution of neuronal activity. Upon hearing the verses of Rubén Darío, complex brain systems start to function, neuronal groups oscillate at 40 Hertz, thalamic-cortical links are established, connections inside each hemisphere are activated, the two hemispheres communicate with each other through the corpus callosum, and excitatory or inhibitory neurotransmitters are emitted. The brain understands the syntactic structures and the meanings of words. It is obvious that information is stored in the nervous system that, in addition to enabling the literal comprehension of the verses, generates a cascade of associations, some of which the writer certainly looked for intentionally: the sky, joy, and that which is precious coming out of the immense blue, the gleeful cloudage and the gold dust. But whoever hears the poem will add personal associations with the scent of loved ones, longed-for desires, or the nostalgia of a foggy day in Paris. Here is where what Changeux calls the pre-representations corresponding to dynamic, spontaneous, and transitory activity of the neuronal groups capable of forming multiple combinations operate.[18]

Although the experience of blue that Darío's verses evoke has an obvious cultural base, even here, we can find innate traces in color perception. When blue is associated with yellow golden dust we are faced with a contradictory situation: our brain is incapable of imagining reflected light that is simultaneously blue and yellow. We are not capable of seeing bluish yellow or yellowish blue. Nor can we identify colors that are both greenish and reddish at the same time; and in contrast we do see the mixture of blue and red as purple or yellow and red as orange. Of course, there is no physical, cultural, or logical reason that prevents seeing the two pairs of opposite colors simultaneously. The wavelength is a continuous phenomenon; there is no cultural taboo that prohibits such combinations nor are there formal impediments. The trichromatic photoreceptor cone system in the retina explains coding in three basic colors (blue, green, and red), but it does not enable comprehension of the wide and variable spectrum of cultural categories that give names to the colors. Nor does it explain what prohibits combinations of red with green or blue with yellow. To do this it is necessary to take into account Ewald Hering's theory that states that in certain areas of the retina neurons produce two pairs of opposite chromatic signals (red/green, blue/yellow) and a pair of achromatic signals (dark/light). Other factors that have an impact on color appreciation would have to be added: their appearance changes, depending on the contrast with contour peculiarities, according to their adaptation to backgrounds, and due to the influence of environmental lighting. Visual information is sent from the retina to the lateral

---

[18] Changeux, *L'homme de vérité*, p. 93.

geniculate nucleus and from there to the primary visual cortex by way of three pathways: the parvocellular, the magnocellular, and the koniocellular. The information is encoded and distributed in a very complex manner; and it is not known if the principal functions of color interpretation are produced during the flow from the retina to the cortex or if they are localized in a cortical center specialized in chromatic information.[19]

Although Darío's verses mainly evoke visual images, there is also a reference to scents. It is believed that in the course of evolution, the importance of color vision provoked the decrease of olfactory functions in the brain. Odor encoding is similar to that of colors. Around one thousand olfactory receptors capable of being activated by different smells have been discovered. Each receptor is fabricated by a specific gene, recognizes the molecules of just one aroma, and sends the information directly to the olfactory bulb in the brain. Nasal epithelial cells that have the same receptor all send signals to the same glomerulus in the olfactory bulb (there are two glomeruli per receptor, in other words, two thousand). The smells that we can recognize and name are the combination of signals sent by hundreds of receptors. And so, the olfactory system encodes about one thousand smells and can recognize some ten thousand particular combinations. This means that, as in the visual system, from the transduction process, when sensory neurons send chemical and electrical signals as a response to external stimuli, we find an encoding process that separates and marks the molecular or luminic information.[20] It should be emphasized that the same thing does not take place in the auditory system that perceives sound wave frequencies: no segmentation takes place there, so we hear the entire sequence of tones, from the highest to the lowest, without interruptions. Tone encoding apparently has an entirely cultural origin.

I wish to stress that if we proceed from the hypothesis of the exocerebrum, we can observe a *continuum* in the consciousness of blue that joins poetic symbols, their linguistic expressions, chromatic images, excitatory and inhibitory reactions, cortical connections, associations, and motor and emotional responses. The consciousness of blue is a continuous coming and going along circuits that are at the same time cultural and neuronal, external and internal, social and private, symbolic and signal-related, mental and corporeal.

Consciousness, of course, is not only the brief flash that enables us to become aware of the conglomerate of metaphors and images contained in the verses of Darío. It is the prolonged and coherent flow – as understood by William James – that gives us unity as individuals and provides us with a keen sensation of identity. However, for the purpose of this reflection, I have only taken into

---

[19] Wandell, "Computational neuroimaging."
[20] Axel and Buck, "A novel multigene family may encode odorant receptors." The authors received the Nobel Prize in 2004 for this research.

account the small fragment of consciousness that is revealed when we listen to these verses of Darío. My proposal is that the nineteen words that make up the four verses, their syntactic links, their rhythms and their rhyme, the swarm of visual images that they evoke, and the communication with the person who reads them out loud *are part of consciousness*, a part intimately connected with memory, with linguistic resources housed in the brain, and with emotional circuits that are excited. The consciousness of blue is an articulated and interconnected swarm of neuronal and cultural instances whose coherence and continuity allows this particular experience. I believe the brilliant intelligence of Helen Keller allowed that blind and deaf woman to intuit the presence of an exocerebrum that helped her, so to speak, to *see* and *hear* those aspects that her senses did not perceive. What she did not look at she managed to see; what she did not listen to she managed to hear. How? She explains it herself when, upset, she criticizes those who think that the blind and deaf do not have the moral right to refer to beauty, the skies, mountains, the song of birds, and colors: "And nevertheless a daring spirit pushed me to use words about vision and sound whose meaning I can guess only thanks to analogies and fantasies."[21] Helen Keller's moving grievance against those who assume that blindness and deafness isolate her from the things others can enjoy is very symptomatic. She argues that a large part of the pleasures in daily life come from the dangerous game of imagining analogies and from the enormous power of touch, smell, and taste that she has developed. She mobilizes a powerful symbolic substitution system that lets her artificially build, in the dark and silent hollows of her exocerebral networks, the chromatic and musical sensations she is lacking. She had such a vast culture and such a penetrating intelligence that she was capable of understanding the prosthetic nature of the exocerebrum and of managing it with great ability to repair and balance her consciousness of the world, at the same time that she was building her identity: "When we consider," she answers her critics, "how little has been found out about the mind, is it not amazing that any one should presume to define what one can know or cannot know? I admit that there are innumerable marvels in the visible universe unguessed by me. Likewise, oh confident critic, there are a myriad sensations perceived by me of which you do not dream."[22] She, more than the majority, thanks to her terrible deficiencies, was able to recognize the symbolic prostheses in culture that enabled her to substitute auditory and optical sensations. It is not very different from what we do when we hear the verses of Darío, which are like a prosthesis that we lean on to understand and to feel that the immensity of blue can become clouded by the scented and dreamlike pleasure of golden dust.

[21] Keller, *The world I live in*, pp. 28–29.   [22] *Ibid.*, p. 29.

11   The musical spheres of consciousness

As we have seen, one of the greatest difficulties in understanding the relation between neuronal circuits and cultural networks is the rather rigid nature of linguistic codes, of the semantic system of meanings, and of syntactic structures. It is not easy to find neuronal correlates that reflect the peculiarities of speech. But if we jump to another cultural ambit, where symbols are very flexible and meanings lack a conventional fixation, perhaps we can obtain a different and illuminating approximation to the question of self-consciousness. I am referring to musical expressions that I have previously mentioned with regard to the theories of Susanne Langer. Just citing the concept, musical "expressions," puts us in front of a complex situation. I will refer principally to the so-called classical instrumental music that is not accompanied by words. For centuries it has been said that music, composers, and performers "express" different emotions, passions, moods, and frames of mind. Of course this idea presupposes that music is able to, in those who listen to it, stir the feelings, excite the emotions, and arouse the affections in such a way that they apparently correspond to the explicit intentions of the creator and the interpreter. Langer, proceeding from the apparent link between the emotions and music, has emphasized that it is necessary to understand that this connection implies a *representation* link with feelings and emotions. That is to say, in music there is a symbolic component that allows for the understanding that emotions are represented in a particular form by sound sequences and combinations. Susanne Langer maintains that there is an isomorphism between emotion and music and that musical representations are inexpressible; in other words, that music reveals states of mind and feelings that cannot be expressed equally as well through language or other symbolic systems. Now, what is the relation between a specific musical form and a specific emotional one? Langer has been criticized for not defining or determining what the *form* of the emotions could be.[1] I cannot give a general answer, but I do propose that it is precisely the structures

---

[1] See Laird Addis's interesting book, *Of mind and music*, which creatively and intelligently develops Susanne Langer's thesis (p. 25 on the "form" of the emotions). It is curious that Arturo Rosenbleuth used the example of Beethoven's piano sonata opus 111 in its different

of music that are one of the forms the emotions acquire – their symbolic form – and they are located in the exocerebrum.

It is well known that since ancient times the Greeks established a connection between certain modes ("harmonies") and specific states of mind. In his *Politics*, Aristotle specifies that melodies imitate character and therefore the Mixolydian mode makes people feel sad, while the Dorian mode moderates temperament, and the Phrygian mode inspires enthusiasm.[2] The modes ("harmonies") of Aristotle and Plato were the tones of the scales of Cleonides and Ptolemy, a combination of note, tone, and type of voice that made reference to regional melodic styles. The essayists of the Renaissance and the Baroque periods maintained theories that linked arrangements with the arousal of feelings and stimulation of emotions, according to intervals and dissonances. This tradition continued through the Enlightenment, embodied in Diderot and Rousseau, and up to the present day. However, it is impossible to think of a dictionary of musical symbols with their corresponding translations in emotional terms. Without a doubt, it is possible to find musical correlates of the emotions, but we would never be able to agree on the definition of tonal sequences and precise rhythms for admiration, anger, hope, melancholy, pride, and vanity. We can conceive of there being emotions that are easily recognized in specific pieces of music, such as happiness and sadness. But it would be very difficult for us to be able to define a musical passage as an expression of envy or shame. And nevertheless, we firmly believe that a composer has imbued the expression of love, anxiety, blame, rejection, obsession, nostalgia, and surprise in his music. But in a dictionary we would not be able to establish emotions, classified alphabetically from admiration to zeal, with the corresponding musical codes that could symbolically represent them. And, even though it has been suggested, it is not possible to confirm that tones are the words, harmony is the grammar, and themes are the syntax of music.

In order to reflect upon the question of the musical form that an emotion, a mood, or a feeling can acquire, I would like to use specific examples. On certain occasions composers have literally referred to a passage or movement with the word *melancholy*. What have they wanted to say? We can suppose that Jean Sibelius wrote his opus 20 for cello and piano, entitled *Malinconia*, to express

---

forms: sheet music (1822), performance (by Schnabel, 1932), and the later impression in a phonographic disc to explain the isomorphism that exists between the messages we receive from the outside world through afferent sensory fibers and the structure of original objects and events. But he does not explain how the isomorphism could continue in the nervous circuits (*Mind and brain*).

[2] *Politics* 1349b, 1–5. Recently, Deryck Cooke, in his book *The language of music*, has tried to establish relations between the twelve-tone scale and the sensations of pleasure, happiness, pain, affliction, desire, etc.

the emotions caused by the death of his youngest daughter from a typhoid epidemic in 1900. It is possible that his pain caused the long, contorted, and insistent piano passages and the intensely dark and even irritating tone of the cello. The melancholy emanating from that piece most certainly perturbs us and carries us into a particular emotional flow. I can imagine a very different situation if we listen to Pyotr Tchaikovsky's *Sérénade mélancolique* (opus 26, from 1875). I believe that here the composer, more than expressing his own melancholy, has the intention of gently awaking that emotion in the listener in such a way that the sadness evokes pleasure and pain, along with abandon. It could be said that Tchaikovsky knows how to manipulate specific melodic sequences that due to their intrinsic character produce melancholy in the listener without necessarily communicating intense suffering on the part of the composer. A third musical experience is found in the final movement of Beethoven's sixth quartet, opus 18, which begins with a gloomy adagio entitled "La Malinconia." It seems to me that in this piece from 1801 the composer did not wish to express his own pain or provoke it in the listener: his intention was to present a simulation of melancholy through distressingly inconclusive sequences alternating with rapid passages that seem like simulations of mania.

Another trio of works that could be successively listened to as *expression*, *provocation*, and *simulation* of melancholy are: *Melankoli* by Edvard Grieg (Lyric Pieces IV for piano, opus 47, no. 5, 1885–6); *Romance oubliée* by Franz Liszt (Andante Malinconico for cello and piano, 1880); and *Melancholic* by Paul Hindemith (first variation of the ballet *The four temperaments*, 1940). We can understand that in regard to different explanations of the musical phenomenon, the forms of expression, provocation, and simulation of emotions implicate some kind of symbolism that allows communication between composers, interpreters, and listeners. In order to put forth my proposal it is not necessary to discuss the causal theories about emotion in music. It is enough to demonstrate that from any perspective in music we find a phenomenon of symbolic interpretation of the emotions and states of mind. However, it is impossible for there to be a conventional classification of the forms of expression, stimulus, or simulation and, consequently, of representation of the emotions. Let us go back to the examples: if we carefully listen to the abovementioned pieces, we will understand that not even a classification in three categories (expression, stimulus, and simulation) is adequate, certain, and stable. If we comment on our impressions with other people we will discover that the interpretation of these pieces is relatively variable and that it also changes depending on the day and hour that we listen to them. Music is not an articulated set of natural signals that, like the aromas of plants or the sounds produced by animals, involves a determining link between what is represented and the representation. Music is located in an imprecise place between natural signals and conventional symbols of speech. Thus, based on Langer's ideas, Laird Addis proposes that music represents certain consciousness states in a "quasi-natural" form. In other words, it would be a necessary emotional expression determined by the peculiarities of our species.[3]

The difference between the conventional symbolic forms of speech and the non-conventional forms of music has its correspondence in the topographic organization of the stimuli in the brain. That arrangement is expressed in the so-called lateralization of the brain – that is to say, in the fact that verbal stimuli excite the left hemisphere more, whereas musical and environmental expressions especially affect the right hemisphere. It has been proved that even from the earliest age there is an advantage in the left ear (that contralaterally sends stimuli to the right hemisphere) in the perception of musical and environmental sounds. This lateralization appears around the age of three months.[4] Recent research has shown that there is a specialization in the hemispheres: the right operates with a system that is much more sensitive to tonal frequencies, while the left houses a more rapid system capable of registering acoustic changes. The right side, better equipped for processing music, would be especially sensitive to the tonal spectrum: in contrast, the left side would be more sensitive to temporal sequences, necessary for distinguishing rapid changes in the pronunciation of many consonants. Of course, these two systems are closely interconnected and function simultaneously. Perhaps the differences are related to the fact that the axons of the neurons in the left hemisphere have more myelin, which facilitates impulse transmission velocity.[5]

Cultural symbology has less strength and a different character in musical representations if we compare it with the syntactic and semantic structures of speech. I do not mean to say that symbols are less important in music, but rather that their presence is expressed with greater elasticity and more fluidly. I believe that music, besides representing internal states of self-consciousness, is itself an external state of consciousness. In other words, that "quasi-natural" state assigned to the tonal sequences and rhythms of music is, more precisely, what I have called the *cerebral character* of certain cultural manifestations: there is a continuity between the internal and the external. It is possible that this cerebral aspect is especially notorious in music, equally or even more importantly than in the plastic representations (painting, sculpture, dance). Laird Addis is correct by concluding that when we listen to music, humors and emotions are *presented* to us and thereby our feelings are affected.[6] It could be said that music is a present, live, and fluid segment of consciousness. In this sense, Susanne Langer's idea is

[3] Addis, *Of mind and music*, p. 36.
[4] Bever, "The nature of cerebral dominance in speech behavior of the child and adult." Kimura, "Speech lateralization in young children as determined by an auditory test." Glanville, Best, and Levenson, "A cardiac measure of cerebral asymmetries in infant auditory perception."
[5] Zatorre and Belin, "Spectral and temporal processing in human auditory cortex."
[6] Addis, *Of mind and music*, p. 112.

tremendously attractive and stimulating: "there are certain aspects of the
so-called 'inner life' – physical or mental – which have formal properties similar
to those of music – patterns of motion and rest, of tension and release, of
agreement and disagreement, preparation, fulfillment, excitation, sudden
change, etc."[7] I would add repetition, a structural element of music that has
different modalities: by sections, by variations, by fugal treatment, and by
development. It is interesting to imagine that nervous activity adopts forms
that are similar to the round, the chaconne, the fugue, the motet, or the sonata.

In a certain way the idea that there is a correspondence or a connection between
music and the internal processes is very old. In *Timaeus*, Plato explains that the
harmony of sounds contains movements similar to those of the soul, although he
warns that the characteristic revolutions of music should not be taken advantage
of for the sake of irrational pleasures, but only as a means of putting in order any
disharmony that could arise in the orbits of the inner spheres. Even Edward
Hanslick, a formalist critic completely opposed to the idea that music can express
emotion, recognizes that it can represent "dynamic properties" of feelings, such
as increasing and decreasing intensities, slowness, speed, weakness, or strength.[8]
Here it is convenient to clarify that, strictly speaking, there is no movement in
music. Nothing is displaced from one point to another in space, but there is,
however, duration, time. The succession of notes, some higher and others lower,
in specific rhythms, is not really movement, but rather the symbol or the metaphor
of movement: "up" or "down" are mere conventions. Certainly it is common to
describe music by associating it with body movements in such a way that we
define certain passages as agitated, peaceful, slow, languid, weak, tranquil, or
funny.[9] From these dynamic references, sadness is usually described through
slow, tranquil music in the lower registers, despite the fact that there are musical
expressions with these characteristics that are not defined as sad, and sad people
do not necessarily speak in a low voice, move slowly, or act tranquilly.

Many philosophers and researchers have come to the conclusion that music is
a cultural phenomenon that is much more closely connected to the body than
other symbolic expressions, such as the fine arts or literature. Speech itself,
produced by the vocal chords, acquires encoded symbolic forms through conventions that are distanced from somatic references. I am interested in the link
between music and the body, because the emotional components of music can
thus be situated in the brain processes that articulate them. To illustrate my idea

---

[7] Langer, *Philosophy in a new key*, p. 228.
[8] Hanslick, *The beautiful in music* [1854], cited by Malcolm Budd, *Music and the emotions*,
p. 22.
[9] See a proposal in Pratt, *The meaning of music*, about the links between body movements and
music. Doubtlessly, the close relation between music and dance – another important expression of
the exocerebrum – has contributed to movements being attributed to different tonal sequences and
rhythms.

I will use, in the form of an experiment, the musical theses of the great philosopher Schopenhauer. For this experiment I will make use of his revealing interpretations of the relation between music and the will, but I will eliminate the metaphysical structure supporting them. Obviously this destroys an essential element of his thought, but on the other hand it lets us observe certain intuitions that arose from his musical sensitivity. I will rely on a few of the interpretations of Schopenhauer's thought made by Malcolm Budd that translate the German philosopher's formulations into terms that are discussed today by music theorists. For Schopenhauer there is an analogy between the temporal sequence that is characteristic of melody and human consciousness. Consciousness connects all its parts into a unified vital flow. Melody, in turn, is a consequence of different tones that are connected in a process that has a beginning and an end, passes through stages that presuppose previous sections, and moves toward a more or less expected continuation. The same thing happens with human conscious life, whose meaning, in a single temporal sequence, unites a past that is connected with an expected future. For Schopenhauer the alternation of dissonances and reconciliations of two elements – rhythm and harmony – is characteristic of melody. On the harmonic plane, melody moves away from the tonic until the moment it reaches a harmonious note: an incomplete satisfaction is produced here from which melody returns to the fundamental note and complete satisfaction is achieved. In order for this to occur, the harmonious moments need to be supported by rhythm that accentuates certain measures. Thus, at specific points harmonic intervals coincide with the accentuated rhythm and move away from it at others, resulting in moments of rest and points of satisfaction.[10]

The succession of consonances and dissonances allows Schopenhauer to establish links between happiness and melodies that pass from desire to satisfaction in rapid cycles. In contrast, sadness is represented by slow melodies that use painful dissonances and last for many measures before returning to the tonic. So in this manner, *allegro maestoso*, with its long passages and changes, assimilates the noble forces directed toward a distant object that is finally reached. An *adagio* refers to the likewise noble suffering that scorns superficial happiness. I do not want to simply return to the unsolvable theme of the encoding of the emotions by means of different types of melodies. What is interesting about this is that once the relation between emotions and melodies is

---

[10] When Schopenhauer speaks of music he is thinking of the melodious operas of Rossini. The Italian composer is an extraordinary model for him because he expresses himself in a pure musical language that does not try to mold itself to words or imitate reality. In contrast, he looked down on the music of Haydn. Would he have realized that, for example, in the *William Tell Overture* we hear an impressive musical description of a storm?

established, Schopenhauer arrives at the conclusion, according to Budd's interpretation, that music is not capable of representing the object of a desire or a
feeling, or their motives, but only those emotional elements that have to do with
will: ease or difficulty, relaxation or tension, satisfaction or desire, pleasure or
pain. Therefore *music is a representation of that which cannot be represented.*[11]
This idea is extraordinarily stimulating to me and helps us formulate the
problem of the relation between a cultural world filled with representations
and a cerebral space that operates through non-representational processes. By
forcing the Schopenhauerian idea of will, which he also saw as an expression of
physical reality, it can be thought of more precisely as a reference to the brain
mechanisms that are intimately tied to the emotions. Antonio Damasio explains
that emotions form part of the homeostatic regulation that assures survival of the
organism, and they form groups of polarized sensation processes oscillating
between positive and negative, pleasure and pain, drawing near to or moving
away from, reward or punishment, advantage and disadvantage. Inspired by
Schopenhauer we could very well say that these oscillations are an expression of
will: essential ingredients of primary emotions such as happiness, sadness, fear,
anger, surprise, and disgust.[12]

Music cannot represent ideas and motives associated with emotions, but
can only represent the sensations of pleasure or displeasure, of satisfaction or
desire. Perhaps the emotional processes that principally implicate the subcortical regions (hypothalamus, brain stem, anterior brain) are found in a
comparable situation: they cannot represent ideas or manage symbols associated with the emotions, but instead they only operate through chemical and
electrical responses that form distinctive patterns of reactions and tensions,
acceptation or rejection, pleasure or displeasure. I ask myself if music can
provide us with the keys for understanding the "will" that drives the neuronal
circuits associated with the emotions. Music would be a symbolic representation of internal emotional states whose neuronal structure lacks strictly representational components.

Perhaps we can compare this paradoxical situation to that strange experiment
carried out by Goethe, which Schopenhauer liked so much: for the representation
of some of his plays, he had organized courtiers who only knew their role, but did
not know the context of the piece until the moment of its public presentation.
Schopenhauer believed that life was a representation of this kind, where the actors
do not know the lines of the others. The cerebral theater of the emotions could be

---

[11] Schopenhauer's ideas on music are expressed in chapter 52 of the first volume of *The world as
will and representation* and in chapter 39 of the complementary volume. See Budd, *Music and
the emotions*, p. 91.
[12] Damasio, *The feeling of what happens*, pp. 50–55. It also takes into account the secondary
"social" emotions such as embarrassment, jealousy, guilt, or pride.

something similar: only when they appear represented on the external public stage do they acquire full meaning. Toward the end of chapter 25 of *The world as will and representation*, dedicated to music, Schopenhauer cites his favorite metaphor once more: the arts, especially music, are like a camera obscura, like a theater within a theater, or a scene within another scene, where objects can be seen with greater purity and at a single glance. The advantage of music over the rest of the arts, Schopenhauer believes, is that while they reproduce only shadows, it represents essences.

It occurred to Antonio Damasio to use the sheet music of a musical piece as a metaphor for the mind. The flows of images, that constitute the internal counterpart of what we observe, are like the different musical parts of orchestral sheet music in the mind, that represent external scenes, objects, feelings, and emotions. He believes, however, that there is a portion of the internal sheet music for which there is no precise external counterpart, and it is that part which goes with the sense of identity characteristic of self-consciousness. Damasio thinks of music as a metaphor only insofar as different melodies and groups of instruments concur to form a coherent internal flow.[13] But it does not occur to him to think that real music that people listen to, besides being a useful metaphor, is also an external prolongation of those increases and decreases in the transmitting chemical substance emission of subcortical neurons and that they are associated with sensations of acceleration or braking, and of pleasure or displeasure. Musical hallucinations that certain deaf people experience – equivalent to the phantom limbs commented on previously – could indicate that, when the flow of acoustic information is interrupted, brain circuits that convert simple sounds into complex patterns look for music in the memory and process it as if it had come from the outside. In some individuals, due to the lack of necessary stimuli coming from the exterior, internal circuits would make their own phantasmal prosthesis.[14]

Damasio himself writes that "sadness consistently activates the ventromedial prefrontal cortex, hypothalamus and brain stem, while anger or fear activates neither the prefrontal cortex nor hypothalamus."[15] Without a doubt, the emotions produce "noises" and signals in the brain that have just begun to be deciphered. Neuroscientists are now listening to a concert of synchronies, discords, periodic oscillation frequencies, neuronal firing velocities, transmitting substances that inhibit or stimulate, and modulations of variable intensity.

The possibility that an exocerebral prolongation of neuronal processes tied to the emotions is contained inside music can be explored if we try to find elements in music whose presence is indispensible for understanding it. Are there forms and organizational systems of sound without which listeners cease

---

[13] *Ibid.*, p. 88.   [14] Griffiths, "Musical hallucinosis in acquired deafness."
[15] Damasio, *The feeling of what happens*, p. 61.

to understand music? The problem becomes complicated because it is difficult to find a universal form of organization, and in contrast, we can demonstrate that musical forms of expression have changed significantly in different epochs and cultures. Leonard Bernstein, in an attempt to find a musical equivalent to the generative grammar of Chomsky, proposed the harmonic series as the fundamental universal structure from which the tonal system arises. The harmonic system, which is definitely based on a natural acoustic phenomenon, would not only be the origin of European tonal music, but also of all musical form, whether cultured or popular, symphonic or folkloric, polytonal or microtonal.[16] Of course this affirmation has been questioned. But in addition, with respect to our topic, nothing demonstrates that the harmonic series is encoded in the central nervous system, as Anthony Storr has observed.[17] So where and how can we look for the connection between the flow of expectations and resolutions, which is the base of Schopenhauer's interpretation, and the neuronal circuits?

I would like to address the problem with a historic example: the emergence and development of atonal forms in twentieth-century European music. As we know, Schopenhauer bases his arguments exclusively on the tonal system. The use of the diatonic scale establishes *which* sound is dissonant and how to look for a consonance to resolve it. This determines the expected effect, when we move away from the principal tonality, and therefore the desire to return to the origin. The interplay consists of inviting the tonic to a prediction of a return, a diverted and delayed return, confronted with satisfactory surprises that do not reach the point of breaking the tonal organization.[18] Alessandro Baricco considers that the so-called "new music" annihilates tonal organization: "Suspended in space with no atonal music coordinates, the listener can no longer make predictions. A note, a group of chords, can be followed by any note. The expectation-and-response mechanism that governs the pleasure of the listening experience collapses." The expected event is replaced by a surprise one. But because there is continuous surprise in atonal music, there can be no prediction and the idea of surprise disappears. So Baricco considers that "if nothing can be expected, nothing can surprise, in a strict sense. Thus, for the ear, atonal music is converted into a sequence of simply undecipherable, mute, and strange sonorous events."[19]

---

[16] Bernstein, *The unanswered question*, p. 33.

[17] Storr, *Music and the mind*, especially chapter 3.

[18] This description of consonances and dissonances in diatonic music does not exactly coincide with Schopenhauer's curious theory of the physical bases of harmony which is: when two tones maintain a "rational" relation they are consonances – there is a coincidence in their vibrations – and when there is no coincidence, the tones are dissonant. See Malcolm Budd's commentary on this (*Music and the emotions*, p. 93).

[19] Alessandro Baricco, *L'anima di Hegel e le mucche del Wisconsin*.

This would explain why the public has pulled away from atonal music and why it is only appreciated by small minorities. Baricco himself, however, recognizes an objection: although the new music rejects the tonal system, it uses alternative forms of organization within which the dialectic that contrasts presentiments, hopes, and expectations with replicas, surprises, and resolutions can operate. Perhaps the problem would lie in the education of the public that now will need to learn the new musical structures and their rules. In regard to this, Charles Rosen, in his book on Schoenberg, says: "A dissonance is any musical sound that must be resolved, i.e., followed by a consonance: a consonance is a musical sound that needs no resolution, that can act as the final note, that rounds off a cadence. Which sounds are to be consonances is determined at a given historical moment by the predominant musical style." Then he explains that the definition of consonances has radically changed in different epochs and cultures and concludes that "it is not, therefore, the human ear or nervous system that decides what is a dissonance."[20]

According to this interpretation, the interaction of dissonances and consonances could trigger flows of predictions, delays, and promises interwoven with surprises, satisfactions, and solutions, within any system – tonal or not. Another matter is whether audiences resist understanding new musical forms. Of course, there is also the possibility that, besides the public, the neuronal circuits of the emotions have difficulty in recognizing, for example, the structures of dodecaphonic serial music, where none of the twelve notes of the chromatic scale have priority. If this is the case, the internalization of the serial structures would be essentially a learning problem in which the isomorphism between neuronal spaces and musical flows would not significantly participate. Of course this question cannot presently be answered. Posing the problem allows us to musically imagine the possible exocerebral particularities of different pieces. For example, let us compare two famous sad and disturbing piano pieces, one by Mozart and the other by Schoenberg. Right at the beginning of the *andante cantabile* of the K330 sonata, after the theme, Mozart changes a single note of the chord at two moments: they are dissonances that cause a shock which then dissolves after the impressive melancholic flow. Now let us listen to the *intermezzo* of Schoenberg's Suite opus 25 in which, in a context of unmelodious sadness, we receive the constant Brahmsian lashes of a severe delirium full of startling surprises. From what I have just said, it is obvious that this piano piece by Schoenberg awakens my emotions and strongly attracts me. But it is obvious that throughout the twentieth century, serial music has not been able to attract a large audience and it is foreseeable that a presentation of the Suite opus 25 would attract immensely fewer people than Mozart's K330 sonata. The question

---

[20] Rosen, *Arnold Schoenberg*, pp. 24–25.

is whether this fact signifies much lower exocerebral content (and a consequent greater intellectualization) in serial music, which makes its connection with internal emotional processes difficult, or if it is an essentially cultural problem of atonal music insertion in a society that (still?) does not recognize it as its own. I am inclined to think that the balance between intellectual character and exocerebral content is related to the capacity of different musical structures to manage the Schopenhauerian combination of satisfactions and expectations – predictable surprises – that confronts us with the emotional presence of a state of self-consciousness that produces sound outside of us, in the concert hall, or in electronic reproducers or transmitters. Scant use of the expectation and response dialectic possibly indicates low exocerebral content in specific musical expressions.

I would like to finish by again taking on a broader theme. I have described textures and circuits in a sensory, sentimental, and emotional dimension. This brings up the disquieting question that many neuroscientists ask: how and why does music not only transmit signals, but also provoke sensations? This is a question that is contained in a more general problem: why and how do we enjoy and suffer sensations instead of simply perceiving signals that could activate the necessary brain functions as a response? Stevan Harnad maintains that the study of neuronal sensation correlates does not allow us to explain how and why we feel them and that without this explanation we will never understand the mystery that is consciousness. Precisely, it is very probable that we are not able to explain how and why we have a conscious flow of sensations, simply by understanding the functioning of the neuronal circuits, activated when we listen to music. My proposal is that in order to solve the problem of consciousness and sensations it is necessary to also look outside of the brain spheres. For Stevan Harnad, the idea of looking for explanations in an endo- and exocerebral continuum is a fantasy that encloses us in a hermeneutic house of mirrors.[21]

A revealing approximation lies in the supposition that, for example, a string quartet about death by Darius Milhaud *forms part* of the circuits of consciousness. When we listen to this quartet (number 3) we deeply feel the sensation of sadness and melancholy. Harnad believes I have simply labeled music as part of the consciousness of our sensations, but that this nominal displacement does not explain how the process works or why we are endowed with feelings instead of functionally responding like zombies without feeling anything.[22] After all, from the Darwinian point of view of survival advantages, it is the same whether we

---

[21] I cite Stevan Harnad from an exchange of letters in which we discussed the problem in June, 2005.

[22] The zombie argument is one of those (sometimes stimulating) absurdities that, Francisco Varela states, obsesses Anglo-American cognitive philosophy. See his conversation with Susan Blackmore in the book she dedicates to interviewing different scientists and philosophers: *Conversations on consciousness*, p. 227. Varela understands very well from his neurophenomenological perspective

respond "functionally" or "emotionally." It is not necessary to feel fear in order to run away from a dangerous animal: a set of instructions and signals could efficiently carry out the same life-saving purpose. In contrast, I believe that extending the field of consciousness and sensations is not a simple question of names. Actually, to suppose that music has exocerebral components that form part of consciousness means that we must think of music as something other than *representations* of sensations. Music also offers us symbolic interpretations of how and why we feel.

It could be argued, as Harnad does, that in a world of insensible beings in which there are only acts and elaborations, including exocerebral symbolic circuits, everything would be exactly the same as in another world, ours, in which sensations accompany consciousness. Exocerebral symbolic circuits could efficiently function in a society of insensible zombies. They would listen to music without feeling it or enjoying it, but they could react by emitting all kinds of signals and carrying out actions (smiles, gestures, movements, dances, comments) that would indicate responses with communicative and social functions that are coherent and comprehensible for the group. Harnad therefore believes that the fact that there are symbolic circuits does not explain how and why humans are conscious and have feelings. This objection is based on the (false) idea that cultural circuits lack causal and explicative powers, a lack that would be characteristic of consciousness and sensations. It is an unproved and unsustainable postulate. From clinical experience, neurologists and psychiatrists know that there is a causal connection between music and brain states. Oliver Sacks gives a good example of this in his book *Awakenings*, in which he narrates the case of a seriously ill postencephalitic parkinsonism patient (Frances D.), treated with L-dopa, who came out of her crisis thanks to music: upon listening to it she became unblocked, abandoned her automatic movements, moving fluidly and easily, dancing agilely. Sacks observed this influence of music on numerous patients suffering from Parkinson's disease, Tourette's syndrome, and postencephalitic parkinsonism; he demonstrated how the regulatory effects of music were reflected in the electroencephalograms of the patients: the signals characteristic of stupor and convulsions passing to normal registers while they listened to music or performed a musical piece were recorded. He cites the case of a patient who knew Chopin's music by memory and by merely saying "opus 49" her electroencephalogram immediately changed. Sacks concludes that his studies "show just how closely the physiological and the existential are tied together" – in other words, neuronal circuits and the networks of cultural life.[23]

that consciousness is simultaneously inscribed or embodied in self-organizing sensorimotor processes and embedded in a biological and cultural context (Varela, "The reenchantment of the concrete," p. 329). See also his book written with Thompson and Rosch, *The embodied mind*.

[23] Sacks, *Awakenings*, "The electrical basis of awakenings," p. 331.

However, the question springs to mind: does the hybrid neuronal/cultural character of consciousness circuits help explain the particular fact that sensations exist, in addition to brain functions and signal transmission? I would say that this hybrid aspect helps the subjective particularities of the most complex sensations and especially the emotions to be understood. The fact of not precisely knowing how and why the basic sensations of pleasure and pain emerged at a particular moment in human evolution does not block the study of more complex sensations of satisfaction or disgust that we observe in music. We are facing the fact that here emotions are closely associated with symbols and we can be sure that if these sensations were stripped of symbols they would be completely different. The fact that symbols are added to functions of feeling is what makes consciousness a process that cannot be explained simply through the observation of endocerebral mechanisms. The causal and explicative character of self-consciousness and the feelings on which it is based is explained by the fact that somatic functions join together with symbols. However, it is clear that the mystery of consciousness is not understood through functional explanations in the language of neurobiologists. If we suppose that the language of music attempts to understand the same mystery, we find that it does not offer us an exact explanation either. When facing the problem of consciousness, where biology and culture converge, we realize that we lack a unified theory that can explain the strange connection of symbolic circuits with neuronal networks. It is not only a problem of "correlation" between sensations and symbols and the search for a "translator" that enables there to be communication between one person (the composer) and another (the listener). If the sensation is accompanied with a symbol, it is no longer the same "pure" or "natural" sensation that hypothetically exists before the translation. If upon seeing the color red I am able to give it a name, my sensation is no longer the same as that of a being that lacks language. The "translation" modifies the feeling; it is an integral part of the sensation. It is more obvious in music: there is no original and natural melancholy that is expressed by the musical symbols of a piano sonata. There is no pure melancholy locked up in an inner Cartesian castle of an "I feel therefore I am" that some musical genius would be capable of "translating" in order to communicate it to the external world through the excellence of his or her art. Symbols and sensations coexist in the same space in the musical spheres of consciousness with no need for interpreters and mediations.

12   Artificial memory

We are very accustomed to using enormous libraries, gigantic databases, and immense information deposits that we can access through the Internet. Obviously, these are artificial memories that function as prostheses for supporting and expanding the limitations of our natural capacity to store information inside our heads. Artificial memories, large or small, are the most obvious example of what I have called exocerebral networks. These external memory circuits include all kinds of registers (baptismal, property, civil, etc.), documentary archives, museums, maps, tables, calendars, organizers, chronologies, cemeteries, monuments, commemorative ceremonies, and the abovementioned libraries, databases, and the Internet. The complexity of these prostheses that store the collective memory is overwhelming. It is worth going back to their humble origins in order to look for some of the keys as to how they work. In ancient times, even though writing was already in use, there was a great dependence on oratory and the oral transmission of knowledge. Everything the Greeks wanted to say in a speech they had to remember and to do so they resorted to mnemonics, a set of devices that helped increase the natural capacities of memory. Plato saw writing as a threat to the memorizing abilities of the soul. In *Phaedrus* he refers to the myth of the discoverer of writing, the god Theuth, who was proud of the fact that writing would enable the Egyptians to have better memories. He presented writing as a "recipe for memory and wisdom." When Theuth showed his discovery to Thamus, king of Egypt living in Thebes, the king told him that to the contrary, "if men learn this, it will implant forgetfulness in their souls: they will cease to exercise memory because they rely on that which is written, calling things to remembrance no longer from within themselves but by means of external marks; what you have discovered is recipe not for memory but for reminder."[1] To avoid this false wisdom perhaps one could resort to mnemotechnics, the art of memory, whose invention was attributed to the poet Simonides in the sixth century BCE. The cultivation of artificial memory also used external resources, but its objective was to fix

---

[1] *Phaedrus* 274C–275B. For a commentary on Platonic praise of philosophical dialectics and its superiority with respect to "graphic speech" see Jaeger, *Paideia*, p. 195.

remembrances in the inner memory rather than store them in written texts. In this way the orator could give long speeches or recitations without the necessity of written notes.

The basic mechanism of this artificial memory (whose practice was considered to be a part of rhetoric) consists of establishing an ordered series of places (such as the rooms of a building) and assigning a mark or image to each one of them that is related to what is to be remembered. In this way, by mentally going through the rooms, following a precise route, the marks or signs that remind one of the assigned themes would appear. In addition to a visual architectural model representing a succession of places in a certain order, the marks that were assigned to each space were given great importance. They were meant to be *imagines agentes*, according to the Latin expression in a famous Roman treatise on rhetoric. In other words, active images or marks capable of being fixed in the memory by leaving emotional impressions thanks to their extraordinary, grandiose, incredible, ridiculous, unusual, dishonorable, or base characteristics. These marks were meant to move the emotions by their singular ugliness, exceptional beauty, or surprising nature. The technique consisted of artificially imitating nature, since it was based on the idea that ordinary daily occurrences are usually forgotten, while strange, new, or marvelous events are naturally retained in the memory.[2]

It is rather unsettling that a Roman treatise on rhetoric from the year 85 BCE, reclaiming the ancient Greek tradition, contains *in nuce* the well-known hypothesis of the "somatic marker" proposed by some present-day neurobiologists.[3] The somatic marker is an internal association between emotional situations and certain complex stimuli. The connection involves a somatic mark (positive or negative) that is added to the memory of a specific stimulus, which facilitates rapid decision-making when the stimulus is later repeated. These marks supposedly form part of an internal preference system housed in the prefrontal cortex. The somatic marker hypothesis has been developed principally to explain the importance of the emotions in reasoning and decision-making in neuronal functions. But the hypothesis has wider implications because in addition to describing how certain experiences that are stored in the memory are emotionally "labeled," it proposes an interpretation of the way in which social conventions and ethical norms are "internalized" as marks that assign positive or negative values to experiences. For their part, ancient mnemotechnics proposed to bring about marks in the internal memory, associated with the emotions, through artificial external means, for the purpose of making it easier for memories to be stored in a certain order and then to flow out effortlessly at

[2] *Ad Herennium*, III, xxii, cited by Yates, *The art of memory*, pp. 25–26.
[3] Tranel, Bechara and Damasio, "Decision making and the somatic marker hypothesis." Chapter 8 of *Descartes' error* by Damasio is dedicated to this hypothesis.

the moment of their public expression in orations or speeches. The *imagines agentes* are markers that signal the existence of connecting points between the sociocultural environment and the brain. They indicate that there are channels through which artificial signals capable of modifying brain circuits flow.

Many people endowed with a prodigious memory – and who participate in international competitions – still utilize the ancient mnemotechnics invented by Simonides and praised by Cicero.[4] It seems to me that the efficacy of the method comes from the fact that it is able to "translate" internal sequences of neuronal signals into symbols and vice versa: to convert ordered series of symbols into neuronal marks that function as links to emotions and experiences. How do the neurobiologists of today explain this phenomenon? They tend to resort to Donald Hebb's proposal, based on the idea that the connections between neurons that fire simultaneously are strengthened. With the theory of conditioned reflexes in mind, Hebb presumed that the neurons that are activated when a bell is heard are connected to adjacent neurons that are activated at the same moment the dog (that Pavlov experimented with) is given food. Thus a neuronal circuit that "knows" that a bell and food are related is formed. Something similar could occur in the example given in the ancient Roman treatise on rhetoric that I have cited (*Ad Herennium*). In order for the counsel for the defense in a murder trial to remember a key point of the prosecution he proposes to imagine lamb testicles: the phonetic similarity (*testis* in Latin is *witness*) makes him remember that there were witnesses who saw the crime. This image is part of an ordered sequence in which other symbols appear: a glass (poison) and some clay tablets (a will, indicating the motive of the crime). We can suppose that the neurons that are activated when testicles are thought of are linked to others that fire when it is known there were witnesses at the scene of the crime. A permanent, or at least a long-lasting, link is formed between the "testimonial" and the "testicular" neurons. This is explained by the fact that the simultaneous neuron activation strengthens the synapses that join them.

The problem is that the enzymes and proteins that strengthen or weaken the synapses must be synthesized from specific genes. But what are the signals that activate those genes? The explanation of Douglas Fields, from experiments in his laboratory, is that the strong stimuli that are produced by simultaneous firing of various synapses (or from a single one being activated repeatedly) depolarize the membrane of a nerve cell. The action potential of these firings makes the voltage-sensitive calcium channels open. Calcium ions then interact with the enzymes and proteins that activate a transcription factor (the cAMP response element-binding (or CREB) protein) that, in turn, activates the protein-producing genes that cause the strengthening of the

---

[4] See the report of Spang *et al.*, "Your own hall of memories."

synaptic connections. This means that the nucleus of the neuron directly hears the firings of the cell and upon doing so determines when the synapsis needs to be permanently strengthened so that the memory becomes lasting.[5]

The ancient author of *Ad Herennium* explained that with the method of fixing information in the memory "art will complement nature." In other words, certain cultural mechanisms are converted into supplements or prostheses of cerebral networks. The mnemotechnical process begins by associating words, things, or ideas to two types of visual images since it was considered, as Cicero said, that "the sense of sight is the most acute sense."[6] The first image is a precise locus situated in an architectural construction. The second image is a mark: the figure of a person, a mask, a god, a hero, or an object that produces an emotional impact. If we continue the sequence in modern terms, we would say that the themes, the loci, and the marks activate three different sets of neurons that initiate synchronized firings until they are able to permanently strengthen the synapses that connect the three groups. Although we are still far from being able to decipher the electric and chemical signals that generate interconnected neuronal networks for establishing memory, we can comprehend that mne-monics has had a profound and lasting impact on western culture. The art of memory was a system that connected the cultural world with the internal microcosm. Not only did it open a communication channel: it allowed for the spheres of the soul to be manipulated by cultural devices. Of course this forced intromission of the powers of the imagination into the elevated rational parts of the soul was a challenge for Christian Scholasticism. Albertus Magnus and Thomas Aquinas, with the help of Aristotelian philosophy, were able to justify the manipulation of images characteristic of artificial memory. The mediating imagery with strong emotional impacts (*imagines agentes*) was substituted by "corporal similarities," which were legitimized by the fact that human cognition is more powerful in the presence of rational things. This played an important role in very subtle and spiritual themes being best remembered in the soul as corporeal forms. Frances Yates has dedicated a marvelous book to the history of artificial memory and has described how this age-old art culminated in Renaissance thought. In my opinion, Yates' book demonstrates that the exal-tation of the art of memory was, among other things, a search for translating apparatuses: of devices to transform ideas into signals capable of immersing themselves into the internal microworld of memory and reorganizing the powers of the soul.

The analysis of Giordano Bruno's thought is one of the most fascinating passages of Yates' work. It is a magnificent example of the obsession to under-stand and perfect the art of memory as a mediating and translating apparatus. It

---

[5] Fields, "Making memories stick."
[6] *De oratore*, II, LXXXVI, 351–354, cited by Yates, *The art of memory*, p. 19.

should come as no surprise that Bruno, in this task of deciphering and manipulating symbols, metaphors, and signs, uses some of the resources that the culture of his time made available to him: cabalism, hermetics, magic, and astrology. He used the images of stars and planets as markers, thinking of them as "superior agents" and placed them in the center of a system of concentric circles (each one with 150 images), conceived as a strange combinatory mediation connecting the celestial spheres with the internal wheels of memory. The images of the stars are connected, in the next circle, to symbols of vegetables, animals, stones, metals, and various other objects. The circle after that consists of a varied list of adjectives, all written in the accusative case. The following circles are made up of a list of inventions (agriculture, surgery, flute, sphere, etc.) with their corresponding inventors (Osiris, Chiron, Marsyas, Atlas, etc.). Frances Yates discovered that Bruno's series of images form part of a system of combinatorial circles like the one created by Ramon Llull. Giordano Bruno built a mediating mechanism that, by manipulating the images of the stars (that are actually "shadows of ideas"), allowed for the adapted images of the "superior agents" to be printed in the memory by means of the concentric circles.[7] As Yates points out, the Renaissance concepts of an animate cosmos such as Bruno's, paved the way for the modern idea of a mechanical universe based on mathematical processes, such as the one Leibniz explored. But Bruno was more interested in the internal mechanics and functioning of the wheels of memory than he was in the external world.

For a vivid and precise idea of the meaning of this mnemonic machinery, one has only to read the beautiful book by the great psychologist A. R. Luria about the case of a man who, because of marked synesthesia, had an absolutely exceptional memory.[8] This person spontaneously associated visual images, flavors, colors, tones, numbers, and words, which enabled him to mentally build spaces, places, and itineraries that were related to the sequences of texts and series of words or numbers that he wished to memorize. But this is not a case of artificial memory: this person took advantage of his "natural" synesthetic condition – the abnormality with which he was born – to carry out the connections and translations characteristic of mnemotechnics in his mind. His synesthesia caused a type of porosity between different brain circuits, in such a way that images, flavors, words, and sounds were filtered, generating stable and lasting associations. A tragic dimension of this extraordinary memorist described by Luria was that the membrane separating him from external reality also had filtrations and so it was often difficult for him to distinguish between real and mnemonic flows.

---

[7] Yates, *The art of memory*, p. 213.

[8] Luria, *The mind of a mnemonist*, originally published by the University of Moscow in 1968. Also see Luria's *The neuropsychology of memory*.

This brief digression into artificial memory has served to be a reminder of, and to stress the importance of, a distinctive link between internal and external marks. The functioning of memory, without artificial intromissions, is doubtlessly a permanent flow of sensations that the nervous system registers and marks non-stop, even though the majority of marks are ephemeral. These passing marks, associated with short-term memory, do not create new synapses, but only strengthen already existing connections. Short-term memory holds memories for seconds or minutes, at the most for a few hours.[9] We can evoke the meaning of this memory with the tragic example of injured people who have lost their long-term memory (which retains memories for days, weeks, or years). Damasio relates the case of one of his patients who suffers from extreme amnesia, whose memory is limited to a small temporal space of less than a minute: once this lapse of time passes, everything witnessed and heard is forgotten.[10] This person remembers very few things about his life; although he recognizes his name and those of his family, he does not identify their voices or their appearance. He is capable of holding a conversation, obeying certain rules of etiquette, and walking along the street. His amnesia was caused by severe encephalitis, which extensively damaged both temporal regions (including the hippocampus and the amygdala). Even though this person lives only in a present that flickers in his brain for a few seconds and then disappears, Damasio says he has what he calls a core consciousness; that is to say, he is aware of an external reality. But he lacks an extended consciousness that implies a self-consciousness and, of course, a long-term memory. Therefore Damasio deduces that the damaged brain regions, that include the hippocampus and parts of the temporal zones, are not necessary for nuclear consciousness. Self-consciousness, however, needs the massive flow of sensations to be filtered so that a part is "filed" in long-term memory.

And this is where the most thorny interpretation problems begin. If the images filed in the memory have to be used consciously, how is it known in which part of the brain to look for them? If we suppose they are marked or labeled, we come up against the Cartesian curse: someone or something – a homunculus – must be capable of reading the marks or labels and extracting the content from each brain file. But we hurl ourselves into the abyss of an infinite regression, since the homunculus or searching agent must, in turn, have a memory that files the necessary codes for recognizing and deciphering marks and labels. If a group of neurons joined by potentiated synapses during the process of reception houses an image, it is possible that there is a chemical mark that labels it (and associates it with other images or emotions). But then there

---

[9] Martin, Bartsch, Bailey and Kandel, "Molecular mechanisms underlying learning-related long lasting synaptic plasticity."

[10] Damasio, *The feeling of what happens*, pp. 113ff.

must be a neuronal system that files the data and keys of these marks. And, in turn, this system must contain marks by which it can be recognized: marks or labels that must then be kept in another group. And this successively continues into infinity. In addition, it still is not known how filed memories are kept, certainly not in the same way as photographic images and phonographic recordings in a realistic movie are. Our homunculus must not only be capable of recognizing labels and marks, but also of deciphering the codes in which memories are encrypted. Neurobiology has not yet found the keys that explain how memory is preserved, nor has it been able to solve the problem of the infinite regression, implicated by the proposal of markers and labels in the brain circuits.[11]

A brilliant study on the metaphors that have been used historically to define memory, written by Douwe Draaisma, has shown that none of them – from the Platonic wax tablet to computers – has managed to escape the curse of the Cartesian homunculus. Neither the wax tablet nor its modern form, the phonographic disc, resolves the paradox: both require an agent that remembers what is imprinted there and how to find it. A computer endowed with neuro-optic exploration mechanisms and programs can recognize visual patterns by automatically comparing them with its own memory, without the need of an additional agent that remembers where the images are kept. However, in the construction of the machine's memory there have been external human agents that have assigned thresholds and limits allowing the machine, for example, to attempt to distinguish (almost always unsuccessfully) a telephone post from a tree. The computer is not capable of recognizing meanings. When a computer recognizes a representation, it is able to do so because meanings have been assigned from the outside.[12]

Now I wish to ask: does the hypothesis of the exocerebrum help us break the vicious circle of infinite regression? Apparently all explanations and metaphors of memory require an *other* (homunculus or agent) to decipher the neuronal marks. The problem is that, as far as is known, there is no one or nothing inside the brain that can carry out this function. In contrast, outside the brain there are a multitude of *others*, homunculi and agents, capable of helping with these recognition tasks. I am referring, of course, to the exocerebral networks that are extended throughout society and that include the immense resources of artificial memories. This interpretation, certainly, implies that the processes that

---

[11] Research on neuronal codes corresponding to sensory stimuli is very complex, since cognitive tasks include different regions of the cortex. A study of the processes of discrimination of different stimuli as the basis of decision-making, carried out in monkeys, indicates that neuronal encoding of the number of firings is more important than the regularity of time intervals between each firing. This study presents an even balance between advances and obstacles in the study of neuronal encoding: see Romo, Hernández and Salinas, "Neurobiología de la toma de decisiones."

[12] Draaisma, *Metaphors of memory*, p. 227.

enable the recording of filed information in the cerebral memory can only function fully if external cultural circuits are utilized. There is a system of marks, signals, symbols, and references in these external circuits that guides neuronal activity in localizing data in the internal memory. This mnemonic exocerebrum, which is much more than a data depository, is formed by a dense network of social connections that, through all kinds of stimuli, renews memories in a permanent flow. The process of remembering the image of a person who is a friend, for example, is not only the work of solitary introspection. There are always social and cultural marks, signals, and stimuli that trigger and support memory recuperation. And I am not only referring to the obvious relation between memory access and seeing a photograph or mentioning the name of the person, but also to a multitude of elements from the daily environment that foster the restoration of memories, without an obvious relation to them. These memories, linked to the image of the friend, are part of a rapid and massive permanent flow of external signals in which there is an important contingent dimension: there is always a combinatorial randomness of stimuli and sensations that makes sure that memories are not always the same and that in turn modifies the memory files. A great number of objects, faces, sounds, words, dialogues, colors, and signs in the spaces that surround us (home, street, office, landscape) form an indispensable network of symbols without which it would be very difficult for us to be able to extensively and efficiently use neuronal memory resources to recover the images of our friend.

This delicate network of mnemonic marks and references goes by relatively unnoticed. It is not as evident as the neighborhood libraries, photo albums, or family chests filled with keepsakes. These subtle textures that surround us are not as spectacular and coherent as the imposing artificial memories that store the history of a civilization, but without them the brain circuits would dry up, and memories would tend to break apart and to adopt strange forms. We can imagine what a mental landscape of a memory devoid of the subtle daily exocerebral networks would be like if we evoke what happens in dreams, when consciousness is turned off and we are disconnected from our surrounding reality. The memories, images, and emotions emanating from the internal memory are grouped into oneiric flows unguided by exocerebral marks. They are not chaotic and disorderly flows, but they follow the courses of a strange logic dominated by a phantasmal exocerebrum that substitutes the external symbolic fabric that, when we are awake, contributes to giving form to consciousness.

A distinction is usually made between two kinds of memory – explicit and implicit. The former is a long-term memory that could be compared with artificial memories that are organized to operate coherently and permanently (archives, libraries). Implicit neuronal memories are those that in a relatively unconscious manner accumulate habits, abilities, representations, conditionings, or repetition mechanisms that have been learned and that can be activated "automatically" and "rigidly." It could be interesting to propose the hypothesis that neuronal mechanisms of explicit memory are closely tied to the exocerebrum, while implicit memories (also called non-declarative) can function with greater independence using afferent sensations as modulators of a learned process that functions inflexibly and that does not require consciousness (such as when we drive a car). Different studies indicate that these two forms of memory are based on distinct neuronal recovery processes that are located in different brain zones. Explicit memory is open to new events and to intentional or conscious memory recovery efforts. Its neuronal base depends on structures located in the medial temporal lobe, including the hippocampus and diencephalic nuclei.[13] Whichever way neuronal mechanisms of memory function, it appears that some memory recovery processes are more closely linked to external signs, marks, and sensations than others.

Many neurobiologists are unsettled and even bothered by the apparent dualism implicated in the interpretation of memory as a brain system that needs to resort to external circuits in order to function normally. However, the strictly monistic interpretations that maintain that consciousness (or the mind) is made up only of brain processes have not been able to provide a satisfactory explanation. As a consequence, dualism could seem to be an unavoidable alternative. One of its scientific expressions has been the proposal that consciousness is formed by programs (*software*) that operate in the brain, which would be the equivalent of the machine (*hardware*). Following this line of thought, memory, as an essential part of consciousness, would be *information*, as described by Norbert Wiener, deposited in neuronal networks (that are based on processes that can be explained in terms of matter and energy). That would not be an abandonment of materialism since, according to Wiener's famous expression, the priority of information over matter and energy is a principle without which it would be impossible for any materialism today to survive.[14] I would like to cite a curious and daring theory that has come out of this dualist materialism. Rupert Sheldrake, a British biochemist, believes that brain circuits can be syntonized or associated with what he calls "morphic fields," which are a type of collective natural memory; like gravitational or electromagnetic fields, they are non-material regions of influence located inside and around the systems they organize.[15] Sheldrake's hypothesis is an escape from the vicious circle to the degree that it involves extrasomatic connections, since it supposes that parts of the brain are associated with morphic fields that shape human mnemonic activity. This lets him explain the mysterious phenomena of telepathy, extrasensory perception, or remembrances of past lives, which

---

[13] Squire and Knowlton, "The medial temporal lobe, the hippocampus, and the memory systems in the brain."

[14] Wiener, *Cybernetics*, p. 132.   [15] Sheldrake, *The presence of the past*, p. xvii.

according to Sheldrake would be ways of syntonizing with nonmaterial morphic fields that allow communication through resonances with far away people or the dead.[16] I have given the example of this hypothesis, despite its somewhat esoteric appearance, because it seems symptomatic of the need many scientists feel to jump the somatic barriers of consciousness and the mind. If we substitute morphic fields with symbolic cultural networks, I believe we will find ways out of the problem of the relation between consciousness and the brain and between memory and neuronal functions, that are perhaps more modest, but more realistic. Sheldrake's hypothesis seems to be a response to those who believe that the causal force of consciousness (and culture) could only be explained by a fifth force field in the universe, adding it to the four already known (gravitational, electromagnetic, the two subatomic particle fields associated with weak and strong interactions).[17] Rather than looking for cosmic explanations, I prefer precise scientific research on the relationship between the field of brain circuits and the space of symbolic networks that surrounds people.

I do not think the proposal that there are external symbolic networks is an escape toward a dualist explanation. Actually this idea contributes to the abandonment of the old nature/culture dualism that has made the study of consciousness so difficult. I believe it is about extracting new paradigms from the facts revealed to us by research. Let us look at an example. The presence of external circuits that complete brain functions can be observed in the symbolic processes that allow for the connection between brain hemispheres. The study of interhemispheric connections produces significant indications related to memory and markers (somatic and symbolic). These connections are formed by the corpus callosum and the anterior commissure, a mass of 200 million axons that join neurons from both sides of the brain together. In view of the proven fact that there are very different cognitive processes in each hemisphere, some scientists believe that consciousness can be divided in two. The classic example of this dissection is that of people who have undergone surgery that has destroyed the connections between both hemispheres. This operation is carried out in severe cases of epilepsy that cannot be controlled any other way, and consists of cutting the corpus callosum to keep the abnormal electrical activity from propagating from one hemisphere to the other, causing generalized seizures.

---

[16] *Ibid.*, pp. 220ff. Sheldrake's explanations are more interesting and stimulating than they might seem; they have provoked sharp controversies and have been accused of bringing magic elements into science. I cannot make a scientific judgment about his proposal, but I am able to see that in the area of human culture my hypothesis of the exocerebrum explains things better than the idea of morphic fields of influence and resonance.

[17] This is what Stevan Harnad demands of John Searle (http://eprints.ecs.soton.ac.uk/11007) if he wishes to solve the problem of the mind/brain relation: that feelings, the basis of consciousness, be a fifth independent causal force in the universe.

The first thing observed in these patients, once they have recovered from the surgery, is that – surprisingly – they behave exactly as they did before the operation. They speak and interact normally and have full use of their senses. However, the careful investigations of Roger Sperry, together with his collaborators and students, showed that this normalcy appears to hide the presence of two independently acting minds. In different experiments that separated information transmitted to each hemisphere, they confirmed that in the majority of cases verbal ability came from the left side and that the other side did not have access to linguistic mechanisms. He concluded that the dominant left hemisphere is the one in charge of interpreting actions and conduct through speech. Sensations received by the right eye or hand (and that arrive at the left hemisphere) could be named by the patients that had been operated on. In contrast, they could not name objects (they said they perceived nothing) shown only to the right hemisphere. However, they could non-verbally signal what had been shown to them on the left side and that therefore only the right hemisphere had perceived: with the left hand, they were able to correctly point to an object that they verbally denied having seen or touched. Sperry, who received the Nobel Prize for his discoveries, describes the situation as follows: "Each hemisphere seems to have its own private sensations; its own perceptions; its own concepts; and its own impulses to act, with related volitional, cognitive, and learning experiences. Following surgery each hemisphere also has thereafter its own separate chain of memories that are rendered inaccessible to the recall processes of the other."[18]

This is just one side of the coin: surgical separation reveals the existence of very different processes in each hemisphere. But on the other hand, we see the extraordinary normalcy with which these people can live and behave in daily life, without presenting signs of a split consciousness or identity. How is this paradox to be understood? The explanation that comes up is revealing: the brain hemispheres have two channels for communicating with each other, an internal and an external one. In these patients the first channel – the corpus callosum – has been sectioned. But the second channel – the exocerebral networks – continues to function and does not let these people bump into objects located in the left half of their visual field, stop perceiving and understanding social relations, or get lost or disoriented when receiving acoustic or visual information. The exocerebrum establishes a communication between the hemispheres that permits normal conduct and ensures the unity of their consciousness.[19] But

---

[18] Sperry, "Hemisphere deconnection and unity in conscious awareness," p. 724.

[19] There are those who, based on the case of the divided brains, jump to the conclusion that the unified "I" is an illusion. Since the left hemisphere gives a coherent but false explanation without the opposite hemisphere realizing it, they suppose that it is improbable that consciousness resides in a part of the brain with such a propensity to produce fictions and narratives (verbal) that are not

not everything with these people is normal. In addition to when one hand occasionally does the opposite of the other (one buttons a shirt while the other unbuttons it), important memory deficiencies have been reported. It has been suggested that this decline in the functions of remembering could be related to communication and linkage difficulties.[20] In other words, the mnemonic markers of the exocerebral space are not able to establish adequate bridges with the internal somatic markers, which in many cases require the combined collaboration of distinct circuits (emotional, verbal, pictorial, or auditory) that are found in opposite hemispheres in order to become fixed.

The idea that the exocerebrum is a bridge between brain hemispheres does not imply a dualist interpretation. This bridge is part of a continuous neuro-cultural process whose characteristics and mechanisms need to be studied. We are not dealing with external computer networks plugged into the *hardware* of nerve wiring. Information circulates all along the neurocultural continuum and there is a material *hardware* that consumes energy inside, as well as outside, the brain. The fact that we are dealing with a continuous circuit does not mean that it is homogeneous: obviously there are important differences in the processes contained in it. These processes need to be distinguished, but not by reducing them to a schematic duality with very limited explanatory power.

necessarily true (Damasio, *The feeling of what happens*, p. 187). But consciousness is precisely the affirmation of a highly symbolic and constructed truth that is not the "objective" reflex of a physical reality.

[20] Baynes and Gazzaniga, "Consciousness, introspection, and the split-brain," p. 1358.

13   The lost soul

Very many people, especially if they have religious inclinations, resist the belief that their affections and feelings are merely a property of the nervous system. They have difficulty accepting that consciousness is a biological peculiarity of the brain, the same way that digestion is a biological characteristic of the digestive tract, to use the expression of the philosopher John Searle.[1] It is difficult for even non-religious people to accept that consciousness is the whole of organic processes belonging to a perishable encephalic mass. Of course, one of the main quandaries lies in the fact that the affirmation that consciousness does not exist outside of the brain is equivalent to accepting that there is nothing after death.

It should be recognized that people are right when they intuit that biological processes, alone, do not explain consciousness. However, looking to the religious belief in an immortal soul to explain consciousness does not solve the problem, but rather is an escape from it. Perhaps it placates the melancholy that is born from the thought that identity that is lived in the present, lacks a future once life is lost. But the intuition that there must be processes or dimensions outside of the brain that help explain the phenomenon of consciousness should not be discarded as a metaphysical vision lacking scientific rigor, as I explain throughout this book. I have searched for exocerebral resources in the cultural and social world that aid in understanding the problem of consciousness. Now I would like to refer to a proposal that, without being religious, defends the idea that there is an immaterial world of mental states, conscious and unconscious, which Plato would have defined as "affects of the soul," between the physical and sociocultural world. This is the interpretation defended by the philosopher Karl Popper and the neurobiologist John Eccles in a book that was very much discussed some years ago and that still arouses interest.[2] In this book Popper defends a triadic more than a dualist idea, since he insists in defining an intermediate world between physical states of the brain (World 1) and the sphere of language and social or cultural

---

[1] Searle, *Mind*, pp. 115–116.   [2] Popper and Eccles, *The self and its brain*.

products of thought (World 3). This intermediate world is that of consciousness of the self and of death, with its base in the sensitivity that is characteristic
of animal consciousness (World 2). Unlike his friend Eccles, Popper does not
believe that the second subjective world survives beyond the death of the
individual. Very few scientists today agree with the ideas of Eccles and Popper
since it certainly does not seem necessary or useful to insist on the old
Cartesian ideas that separate the subjective world from its organic bases.
Popper forcibly introduces the second world of sensibility and consciousness
as a kind of mortal soul, but does not succeed in showing that it is actually
nothing more than a configuration of the cultural world based on the brain.
However, it is interesting to observe that Popper recognizes that our personalities and identities "are anchored in all the three worlds, and especially in
World 3." And he adds: "I suggest that a consciousness of self begins to
develop through the medium of other persons: just as we learn to see ourselves
in a mirror, so the child becomes conscious of himself by sensing his reflection
in the mirror of other people's consciousness of himself."[3] In this point,
Popper confesses in a footnote that a friend made him realize that the great
Scottish economist Adam Smith had already said that society is a mirror that
allows the individual to become aware of his character and of the usefulness or
unworthiness of his own feelings.[4] The reader will recall that I began this book
alluding to a similar, but earlier, definition made by John Locke.

The hypotheses of Eccles and Popper, rejected today by the majority of
scientists, contributed to paralyzing the interest in the connections and interactions of the brain with its surroundings since it was feared that this could open
the door to dualism. By opposing (and rightly so) the idea of the second world
(the soul, the psyche), neurobiologists also refused to study the functions of
what Popper called World 3, the world that contains the exocerebrum that I have
been reflecting upon. Even Eccles forgot about this dimension in order to hang
on to a dualism through which he stubbornly tried to demonstrate the existence
of a subjective mental world defined by "psychons" that supposedly modify
brain activity in a way that is analogous to the probability fields of quantum
mechanics.[5]

I have cited the ideas of Popper and Eccles because, in an almost graphic way,
they are an example of the obstacles confronting the search for the exocerebral

---

[3] *Ibid.*, pp. 108 and 110.
[4] Smith, *The theory of moral sentiments* [1759], section 2 of part 3 (or chapter 1 of part 3 in the sixth
and subsequent editions): the chapter entitled "On the principle of self-approbation and self-
disapprobation."
[5] Eccles, *How the self controls its brain*, pp. 81–88. Eccles supposes the existence of a group of
elemental mental events that he calls "psychons" that are linked to fixed anatomical structures; he
wants to calculate the influence of psychons with the Heisenberg uncertainty principle. All this
seems to be a not very interesting attempt to scientifically prove the existence of the soul.

connections of consciousness. If every time we investigate the cultural environment of the brain, the specter of an intervening dimension of a more or less metaphysical nature appears, perhaps we would have to prohibit any search of this kind, unless we were to accept the inevitability of such a spiritual dimension, despite recognizing the impossibility of understanding it from a scientific perspective. In fact, the postulate that there is a particular subjective mental dimension separate from biological and cultural realities is a wall that blocks research and makes us blind. It is as if, let us suppose, before the eyes of a reader of *Madame Bovary*, a thick swarm of spirits, psyches, memes, phenomenical transformers, psychons, translators, interpreters, epiphenomena, or souls would emerge, establishing themselves as the incarnation of an "I" that – with the help of the brain – would be perceiving the erotic melancholy of Emma, the great personality created by Flaubert. I believe that there is actually nothing between the reader's brain and the pages of the novel. Consciousness is simultaneously found in the brain and in the book – not in a metaphysical dimension. The same thing happens when that reader of Flaubert decides to listen to Prokofiev, contemplate a paint by Klimt, or converse with a friend: there is no mediating substance between the individual and what he or she listens to or contemplates. The existence of neurocultural networks does not demand the belief that there is a spiritual space different from nervous textures and social structures. The exocerebrum is not something that is located between the neurons and culture, but rather it is a structured environmental segment that continues certain brain functions by other means.

It might be thought that the exocerebrum is another name for what Michael Gazzaniga defined back in the mid 1980s as the "social brain." But that is not the case. In fact, Gazzaniga's book by the same name is an argumentation about the influxes of brain organization in social and cultural life, and establishes itself as a criticism of those who believe that environmental influence is important in brain development. It also rejects the "externalist" interpretations in which he sees an exaggerated propensity to look for collective social responsibilities when confronting human problems, while for the "internalists" the individual is the responsible entity. He presents things as a type of political confrontation between externalist socialists and internalist liberals. Gazzaniga advises politicians to try to adapt the established order to the nature of the brain and he wishes to do away with the externalist tendencies that he feels haunt us. The conclusion is that the peculiarities of the brain supposedly demand a society that is regulated as little as possible.[6] The "social brain" is a metaphor for describing the central nervous system as a confederation of hundreds or thousands of modules that carry out independent activities in

---

[6] Gazzaniga, *The social brain*, chapter 12.

parallel form. One of these modules, located in the left brain lobe, is the "interpreter" that constructs, so to say, the theory that behaviors of the modules are produced by an "I": in this way the illusion that humans act freely is generated. For this conception the brain is social only to the degree in which a particular image or metaphor of society has been projected onto its architecture.

The great advances in research during the so-called Decade of the Brain have almost totally swept away explanations such as those of Popper and Gazzaniga: scientists have not found traces or signs of the soul either in a spiritual world or in an internal interpreting supermodule that is the unifier of mental functions.[7] However, neurological science, with a strong positivist charge, locked the subject of consciousness in the jail of the cranium and insisted on deciphering the operations of a solitary self – essential and universal – incapable of overstepping the boundaries of factual discourse, like Wittgenstein in his *Tractatus*, that prohibits any and all escape toward the empty spaces of silence that supposedly surround the dominions of language. I have wanted to cite Wittgenstein to show with his example the dead-end of an empiricism that stubbornly imposed limits to exploration. Wittgenstein himself became aware of the problem and in his later studies made a spectacular change of direction by opening the windows of the transcendental self to the huge phenomenological window of cultural experiences. I share the sharp critical dissection that Ernest Gellner has made of Wittgenstein's turnabout, but this is not the place to enter into that prickly subject.[8] I only wish to point out that possibly due to the fact that Wittgenstein realized his errors in the *Tractatus*, he had the intuition that it seems to me pertinent to cite here: "One of the philosophically most dangerous ideas is, curiously, that we think with the head, or in the head. The idea of thinking as a process in the head, in an absolutely closed space, gives it the nature of something occult."[9] Wittgenstein refuses to abandon the idea of the insuperability of the abyss between consciousness and brain processes,[10] and in fact explores the possibility that there may not be a psychophysical parallelism, that there is a causality without physiological mediations, and that it does not mean believing in a vague entity.[11] Giving up the search for psychism's neurophysiological correspondences is absurd and, nevertheless, from these concerns, it occurs to him to suppose that the specifically organic mental process can be "substituted" by an inorganic process that provides a prosthesis for thinking. Wittgenstein asks himself: "How should we have to imagine a

---

[7] In his book from 1998, *The mind's past*, Gazzaniga no longer speaks of modules but he insists on his theory of the fictitious "I" and the "interpreter" located in the left hemisphere.

[8] Gellner, *Language and solitude.*   [9] Wittgenstein, *Zettel*, §§ 605–606.

[10] Wittgenstein, *Philosophische Untersuchungen*, § 412.   [11] Wittgenstein, *Zettel*, § 611.

prosthetic organ of thought?"[12] Even though I read Wittgenstein's proposal after having finished writing this book, it seems to me that I have in some manner answered his question, although in a way that he certainly would not have liked.

The fact that consciousness is not a hidden phenomenon locked up in the cranium and that we can examine its florid arborescent prostheses in the open spaces of cultural life, does not mean that the mysterious halo pervading the subjective sensation that we humans have of being a unique self, irreplaceable and unrepeatable, disappears. I am convinced that science will be able to solve the mystery. Those who declare that if consciousness is a mystery and not a puzzle, then we will never be able to understand it, are wrong. The mysterious – I would say poetic – quality of consciousness does not place it outside the reach of our comprehension. In fact, it was a poet who, through his art, expressed a revealing fact. At the height of an anguished search for his poetic identity, Rimbaud uttered a disconcerting phrase: "Je est un autre."[13] It was referring to the profound immersion of the poet into the world surrounding him. Paradoxically, it is an affirmation of poetic identity that at the same time dissolves the self into the other.

"I is another" – a strange expression that challenges us to reflect. In some mysterious way it expresses the idea that I have presented: consciousness of our individual identity extends to and includes others. The poet reminds us that consciousness is born out of suffering and out of the assimilation of that suffering through the help of others, because we blend with them in order to confirm our transitory identity. In this way we lose the soul but we attain consciousness.

---

[12] *Ibid.*, § 607. He asked himself before: "Is thinking a specific organic process of the mind, so to speak – as it were chewing and digesting in the mind?" See Roland Fischer's stimulating essay "Why the mind is not in the head but in society's connectionist network." He sustains the idea that the mind is found in the interaction between society and individual. The proposal is not developed but it points toward the definition of an individual consciousness as a unit of reproduction in cultural evolution in the same sense that genes are reproduction units of phenotypical organisms.

[13] He repeats the expression in two letters: one from May 13, 1871 to Georges Izambard and one written two days later on May 15 to Paul Demeny. Rimbaud, *Œuvres complètes*, pp. 249–250.

Part II

Brain and free will

14   The hands of Orlac

In the spring of 1924, the premiere of *The Hands of Orlac*, one of the gems of Expressionist film, made such an impression on its Austrian audience that when it was over many of them began to cry out in anger. The lead actor, Conrad Veidt, had to go up on the stage to explain how the filming had been done. The great actor, with his commanding presence and voice, managed to calm the viewers that had been stirred up by the silent film. *The Hands of Orlac* tells the story of a famous concert pianist, Paul Orlac, who loses his hands in a horrific railway accident. A surgeon transplants the hands of a murderer, who has just been decapitated, onto the pianist. Orlac is plagued by the sensation that his transplanted hands are taking over his mind and driving him to commit crimes. His physician explains that he will be able to control the criminal impulses emanating from his new hands by exercising the power of his will. The film is a great dramatic representation of the struggle between the dominating force arising from a part of his body, the hands, and the willpower that must govern the pianist's consciousness. Orlac feels that the hands have taken command of his mind. When his father, whom he hates, is murdered, the pianist is convinced that he was the one who fatally stabbed him, but he has no recollection of the act itself. Apparently, the savage power of the transplanted flesh was capable of directing the mind of the pianist.

The film's director, Robert Wiene, had already created *The Cabinet of Doctor Caligari* in 1920, which was also about a person who was controlled by an assassin. Thanks to hypnosis, a psychiatrist, Caligari, directs the criminal activities of a character who has absolutely no control over his body. But here it is obviously the mind of Dr. Caligari that is capable of determining the behavior of an individual who is functioning like a puppet. In the case of Orlac, it is finally discovered that his own mind has been the unconscious cause of the strange behavior of his hands, because of his certainty that they are the hands of a murderer. When he finds out that the decapitated person, whose hands are now his, actually was innocent, the grafted hands now begin to obey him and the illusion vanishes.

The spectators of that era were confronted with the problem of the opposition between determinism and freedom. Up to what point does the body – and especially the brain – enable consciousness to freely decide? What limits does brain matter impose on the free will of individuals? The problem had political and moral implications, as it does today, because it insinuated that the control of the brain through certain techniques or mechanisms could lead to unconscious irrational behavior. This is precisely what happened during the First World War when the German State sent its citizens into a criminal battle; and as occurred again later, when a large part of the German population was driven to the most despicable attitudes and murderous behaviors.

The hands of Orlac appeared to be impelled by the strange spirit of the assassin to whom they belonged. If we go from the realm of fiction to that of reality, we can approach the question of free will from another angle. The best-known example of obsessive-compulsive disorder is the irresistible mania that drives people to be constantly washing their hands, possessed by the fixed idea that any contact is dangerously contaminating. Everything appears dirty to those afflicted with this disorder. They cannot stop washing their hands after touching a doorknob, money, or a piece of silverware, turning a faucet on, shaking someone's hand, or touching a piece of fabric. They believe that everything around them is contaminated and they live in a constant state of anxiety, fearing they will become infected. The causes of obsessive-compulsive disorder appear to be located in the basal ganglia and the frontal lobe of the brain. At any rate, those affected seem to be dominated by an irresistible force that drives them, even against their will, to behave absurdly; they are usually perfectly aware that they suffer from a disorder that forces them to act irrationally.[1] Other expressions of this disorder make people obsessively collect insignificant objects, excessively check things out of fear that some mechanism or process is not working properly, perform certain actions over and over again, repeatedly and compulsively put things in order, obsessively look for a meaning in numbers they randomly come into contact with, and incessantly evoke the same mental images.

The pathological and abnormal cases strongly underline the presence of a determinist chain of causality. Here the person has not freely elected her or his will to be fettered to biological causes. But we humans assume that under "normal" conditions we are rational beings capable of freely choosing our actions, and so we suppose that there is not enough cause in everything we do to determine our acts. We believe in free will. But there is always a lingering suspicion or fear that the abnormal cases are the ones that will actually reveal the hidden determinist mechanism that, under each and every circumstance, rules us all. This problem, which philosophers have wanted to resolve for many generations, is now being tackled with new tools by the science of neurobiology. The consequences of this new perspective are worth contemplating.

---

[1] See Judith Rapoport's book *The boy who couldn't stop washing*.

Neurobiology has also invaded another terrain traditionally guarded by philosophers: ethics. We can understand that much of modern morality is based on accepting the existence of free will. The notions of sin and guilt are sustained by the supposition that people are capable of freely choosing their actions, making them responsible for the consequences of those acts. Of course, psychiatrists have long outlined an area of behavior that should not be subject to penal considerations (or moral ones) because it is established by a pathological etiology that defines states of mental disturbance. But if we assume that there actually is no free will, we would have to yield to the psychiatrists and neurobiologists and let them look for the mechanisms in the determinist networks that would define moral behavior. What is the cause behind murderous or dirty hands? Is there someone to blame or is there just a causal chain of events? The dirty hands of Orlac or those of the obsessive patient are a metaphor that allows us to situate the problem I wish to examine. When individuals soil their hands – in politics, in finances, in the home – we are faced with an ethical problem. Jean-Paul Sartre, in *Les mains sales*, a play written in 1948 and influenced by the assassination of Trotsky, introduces us to a communist politician who in the view of his comrades has dirtied his hands. They consider him a traitor who has sold out to a class enemy: he is a social democrat, pragmatic, skillful, and a negotiator. His assassin is a young intellectual from a well-to-do family, a hardliner who rejects all alliances with the bourgeois parties. Nevertheless, after the murder, the political line of the reformist leader ends up prevailing in the party, making the homicide incongruous. As it turns out, the assassin acted out of jealousy, having accidentally found the leader kissing his wife. Nonetheless, in the end he takes responsibility for his crime as a political act and lets himself be eliminated by his comrades, who wish to wash away all traces of the horror. The young fanatic dies for a lie.

Here, we face an infinite tangle of causes and effects, a tight network that encompasses psychological as well as social and political processes. Sartre wanted to place the theme of freedom in the context of a succession of contingencies and absurdities. The question that jumps out at us is: can we only escape determinism thanks to the randomness of a senseless life? If a person's life is subject to his or her circumstances, memories, aptitudes, and tendencies, it is difficult to find a space for liberty; it appears to be subject to a determinist structure. But if in order to freely make decisions, the person could be impervious to her or his environment and past, then she or he would live a life subjected to chance. Would it be a life based on freedom or rather on an existence submerged in the absurd? We can suspect that if the determinists are right, not only would there be no liberty: everything would be fate, and as a consequence, there would be no future.

In this second part of the book, I reflect on free will and ethics from the perspective of my hypothesis on the exocerebrum. This means placing the questions of freedom and morality in the terrain of consciousness, understood as a process that links neuronal activity with the symbolic exocerebral networks.

I shall offer an interpretation of the paradoxes and enigmas put forth by ethics and liberty from the viewpoint of my hypothesis on consciousness, defined as part of a symbolic substitution system of functions that the brain cannot carry out exclusively through neuronal mechanisms.

For that purpose I will explore some of the theories that neuroscientists have developed in order to solve the problem of free will. These theories are often based on some variety of determinism and therefore end up negating free will, which they qualify as an illusion. This theme is intimately connected to the philosophical and political discussions on the fundaments of morality. Obviously, if free will is something illusory, there is the danger of undervaluing the entire structure of the social institutions that are based on the belief that it is personal responsibility that makes individuals deserving of punishment if they break the law and of reward if they are sufficiently meritorious. Various neuroscientists have audaciously entered the territories of ethics and morality. I will attempt to bring the reader closer to some of these intellectual adventures so he or she can meditate on the consequences of a determinist vision of the link between the brain and consciousness. This exploration is important because, as will be seen, the determinist interpretation dominates the neurosciences. And it is a theme of pressing importance, given that we are witnessing an explosive expansion of neurological studies in domains that had previously been the private hunting grounds of philosophers, sociologists, historians, anthropologists, or economists. This expansion of the neurosciences should be welcomed because it creatively contributes to erasing the traditional dividing line between the humanities and the natural sciences.

One of the unexpected effects of this extension of the neuroscientific spaces lies in the fact that some neurologists are beginning to realize that the solution to many of the mysteries before them may not be found in their own fields (or only partially). When neuroscientists decided to confront the mysteries of consciousness – that traditionally had been left in the hands of philosophers and social scientists – they began to discover that they could not move about in these new terrains without changing their research strategies. Not all of them accepted the challenge and some merely invaded the new spaces with shortsightedness, not modifying their traditional armamentarium. Determinism has been one of the most critical points of encounter, as well as one of the most abrasive aspects in the relation between humanists and scientists.

In this second part, in addition to discussing the interpretations made by neuroscientists, I attempt to look for answers in little-explored spaces. One of them, which I see as fundamental, is the world of games. I believe that certain keys to understanding free will can be found in play, because it is an activity in which there is a paradoxical mixture of strict rules and the enthusiastic expression of freedom of action. Ludic spaces reveal dimensions that are symptomatic of the functioning of consciousness.

I also wish to explore another dimension that, like play, is intimately close to us. I am referring to the symbolic expressions of the cultural environment that surrounds us. In the first part of this book, I examined some of these manifestations: speech, the arts, music, and artificial memories. Now I intend to take into account other expressions of symbolic substitution systems (or cultural prostheses) that envelop us and crystallize in the home, kinship systems, cooking, and dress. This intimate surrounding world is the closest receptacle in which free will, willpower, and decision-making are expressed. Perhaps it is in this world of small things that are close to us where we can find clues to face the great challenges confronting us when we try to understand the meaning of human liberty.

15   Does free will exist?

In the summer of 1930, Albert Einstein had a revealing discussion with Rabindranath Tagore. The great Bengali mystic was set on finding a space for freedom in the universe, and thought that chance, discovered by physicists at an infinitesimal level, showed that existence is not predetermined. Most certainly, he was referring to Heisenberg's uncertainty principle, also called the indeterminacy principle. Einstein maintained that no fact would allow scientists to dismiss causality; and that the function of order could be understood on the higher plane, whereas this order is not perceptible in minute elements. Tagore interpreted this situation as a contradictory duality situated at the very depths of existence: liberty in conflict with the order of the cosmos. The physicist denied the existence of this contradiction: even the smallest elements maintain an order. Tagore insisted that human existence is eternally renewed due to a harmony that is built upon the opposition between chance and determination. In contrast, Einstein said that everything we do and experience is subject to causality, but he conceded that it is a good thing we cannot see it. To prove his point, Tagore gave the example of the Indian musical system, in which the composer creates a piece that allows for an elasticity expressed by the personality of the interpreter, who then enjoys a certain amount of freedom of interpretation. The discussion moved on to musical themes, because Einstein had a great interest in comparing western music and its rigid patterns with the music of India.[1]

In a letter to the same conversational partner, Einstein made some statements that have been frequently quoted by the determinists. He said that if the Moon possessed consciousness of itself, it would be perfectly convinced that its path around the Earth was the result of a free decision. And he added that a superior being having a perfect intelligence would laugh at the illusion of humans that believe they act according to their free will. Although humans resist being seen as a powerless object subjected to the universal laws of relativity, in fact, their brain functions in the same way inorganic nature does.[2]

---

[1] Tagore, "Three conversations: Tagore Talks with Einstein, with Rolland, and Wells," *Asia*, 31 (3) (March, 1931): 138–143.

[2] Cited by Prigogine, "The rediscovery of value and the opening of economics," p. 63.

The differences between Tagore and Einstein symbolize two great ways to approach the question of freedom. The former, like many religious believers, tried to take advantage of what appeared to be a crack that was opened by the physicists through which the idea of indeterminacy could enter. To many it seemed that the uncertainty principle could somehow mean that electrons were "free" and that they escaped from the causal chain. This vision influenced scientists as important as Eccles, who proposed explaining subjectivity through the presence of "psychons,"[3] as I mentioned in chapter 13.

Einstein's attitude has influenced those who assume that free will, as a property of human consciousness, is a mere illusion. The brain would be crossed by empirically demonstrable causal chains, in which there were a connection between thoughts and actions. The idea that consciousness, acting freely, is the cause of the actions would actually be an illusion. From this perspective, free will is seen merely as a sensation constructed by the organism and not as a direct indication that conscious thought has caused the action, as has been formulated by Daniel Wegner.[4] According to this psychologist, people erroneously believe that the experience of having a will is, in fact, a causal mechanism. Those who believe free will exists are mistaken in the same way as those who thought the sun orbited the Earth. Wegner says that people believed in the Ptolemaic system, in part due to the influence of the religious concepts that placed the Earth at the center of the universe created by God. The belief in a conscious will as a causal agent is a similar error. He recognizes that philosophers and psychologists have spent entire lives trying to reconcile conscious will with mechanical causality. This problem is expressed as a contradistinction between mind and body, between free will and determinism, between mental and physical causality, or between reason and cause. For Wegner, the difficulty lies in the desire to see the world in both manners, which has produced two incompatible ways of thinking. He offers the following solution: "When we apply mental explanations to our own behavior-causation mechanisms, we fall prey to the impression that our conscious will causes our actions. The fact is, we find it enormously seductive to think of ourselves as having minds, and so we are drawn into an intuitive appreciation of our own conscious will."[5] The mind only produces an appearance, a continuous illusion, but in reality it does not know what causes our actions. Inevitably, Wegner turns to Spinoza's famous statement: "Men are mistaken in thinking themselves free; their opinion is made up of consciousness

---

[3] Eccles, *How the self controls its brain*, pp. 81–88. See a comment on this in the first part of this book, chapter 13.

[4] Wegner, *The illusion of conscious will.*

[5] *Ibid.*, p. 26. In a footnote (p. 2) Wegner accepts the fact that qualifying conscious will as "illusion" is a bit strong, and that perhaps it would be more appropriate to qualify it as "construction" or "fabrication." But he uses "illusion" to imply that we put a great erroneous emphasis on how will appears to us and how we assume that this appearance is a deep understanding.

of their own actions, and ignorance of the causes by which they are conditioned. Their idea of freedom, therefore, is simply their ignorance of any cause for their actions."[6]

It is worth pausing to study Spinoza's expression, because viewed out of context, it appears to be the manifestation of an implacable determinism. The phrase comes from the *Ethics*, a marvelous work that Spinoza never saw published and that is, among other things, a powerful call to attain human liberty. How does Spinoza conciliate his recognition of a natural chain of causes and effects with the struggle to achieve true freedom? It is necessary to understand the context and logic from which the quoted phrase is taken. He writes: "Their idea of freedom, therefore, is simply their ignorance of any cause for their actions. As for their saying that human actions depend on the will, this is a mere phrase without any idea to correspond thereto. What the will is, and how it moves the body, they none of them know; those who boast of such knowledge, and feign dwellings and habitations for the soul, are wont to provoke either laughter or disgust."[7] This last line is a harsh reference to Descartes, and the course of reasoning is based on the idea that because humans are ignorant they cannot be free. Previously he has explained that ignorant men believe that all their actions have a purpose that is decided by them and they believe the same in regard to natural events, and therefore end up thinking that the gods direct everything in relation to its usefulness to humans.[8] For Spinoza nature "has no particular goal in view" and he is convinced that all final causes are nothing more than human fabrications.[9] Those who follow a causal chain to find finality in things will never stop asking for the causes of the causes, until they "take refuge in the will of God – in other words, the sanctuary of ignorance."[10]

What Spinoza states is fundamental: in relation to natural acts there is no absolute free will, because that will depends on the understanding of the singular objects that cause the ideas. One must keep in mind that for Spinoza, will is the faculty by which what is true and what is false are affirmed or denied; it is not the desire with which the mind wants things or rejects them.[11] Therefore, "will and understanding are one and the same."[12] This is why he says that there is "no absolute or free will" in the soul or the mind, that "the mind is determined to wish this or that by a cause, which has also been determined by another cause, and this last by another cause, and so on to infinity."[13] It is important to underline that here Spinoza uses the term "free" in the sense of "absolute": as he has said from the beginning of the *Ethics*: "That thing is called free, which exists solely by the necessity of its own nature, and of which the

---

[6] Spinoza, *Ethics*, 2nd part, proposition 35, note.   [7] *Ibid.*   [8] *Ibid.*, 1st part, appendix, c.
[9] *Ibid.*, 1st part, appendix, e.   [10] *Ibid.*, 1st part, appendix, f.
[11] *Ibid.*, 2nd part, proposition 48, note.   [12] *Ibid.*, 2nd part, proposition 49, corollary.
[13] *Ibid.*, 2nd part, proposition 48.

action is determined by itself alone."[14] This is not the case of the mind, which depends on the things surrounding it. He criticizes the Cartesian idea of a soul with absolute power united to a brain thanks to a pineal gland, capable of freely dictating its will to the body.

Let us now take a look at the process that takes Spinoza from denying the freedom of the mind, to exalting the capacity of citizens to act freely. There is no absolute will in the mind, but rather only a set of singular volitions that affirm or deny an idea, for example like the assertion that three angles of a triangle are equal to two right angles. But will is not infinite, it does not extend beyond what we perceive and what we conceive. Spinoza ends the part of his *Ethics* dedicated to nature and the origin of the soul by pointing out how his theory contributes to the practice of living. After advising us to endure both good fortune and bad with a positive attitude and to not hate anyone, he concludes that his doctrine helps individuals to learn to be governed so they may "freely do whatsoever things are best."[15]

Where does the force that can enable humans to be free come from? Spinoza locates that power in what he calls the *conatus*, which is the striving of the mind to persevere in being. The *conatus* is a tendency, propensity, or impulse that includes the mind, as well as the body: "Now as the mind is necessarily conscious of itself through the ideas of the modifications of the body, the mind is therefore conscious of its own endeavour (*conatus*)."[16] He had previously pointed out that "mind and body are one and the same individual thing."[17] Antonio Damasio very correctly has commented that it is fundamental today to restudy the concept of *conatus*, one of the most important keys to Spinoza's thinking.[18] I believe that the idea of *conatus* can be interpreted as consciousness, in the sense of an impulse or effort, based on the body as much as on the social and natural environment, that makes us become self-aware. The possibility of free will lies within this effort. In the fourth part of his *Ethics*, dedicated to human bondage, Spinoza explains that the "free man" is one who lives solely according to the dictates of reason.[19] To advance the understanding and reason of the emotions, we rely on the *conatus* that preserves our identity: "Again, since this effort of the mind wherewith the mind endeavours, in so far as it reasons, to preserve its own being is nothing else but understanding; this effort at understanding is the first and single basis of virtue."[20] Certainly, Spinoza believes that humans rarely live by the dictates of reason. Their helplessness and lack of freedom are determined by the absence of understanding and the weakness of their consciousness. But it is not impossible for them to be led to live "under the guidance of reason, that is, to become

---

[14] *Ibid.*, 1st part, definition 7.   [15] *Ibid.*, 2nd part, final note 1, 4th.
[16] *Ibid.*, 3rd part, proposition 9.   [17] *Ibid.*, 3rd part, proposition 2, note.
[18] Damasio, *Looking for Spinoza*, pp. 170f.   [19] Spinoza, *Ethics*, 4th part, proposition 67.
[20] *Ibid.*, 4th part, proposition 26.

free and to enjoy the life of the blessed."[21] Spinoza describes different virtues and peculiarities of free humans, such as their strength of spirit, the mutual gratitude they show, friendship, and good faith. He adds that "the man, who is guided by reason, is more free in a State, where he lives under a general system of law, than in solitude, where he is independent."[22] He recognizes that human strength is very limited and is surpassed by exterior forces; it must be accepted that we are part of nature and if we understand that clearly, the best of that which is human – defined by intelligence – will come to rest in the natural order of things: "in so far as we have a right understanding of these things, the endeavour of the better part of ourselves is in harmony with the order of nature as a whole."[23]

The fifth and last part of the *Ethics* of Spinoza is dedicated to human freedom and to the power of understanding. It begins with his famous critique of the concepts of Descartes on the relation between the soul and the brain. He finishes up his ideas about the power of the mind over the emotions and his affirmations as to the resulting human freedom. He praises the triumph of wisdom over ignorance, which is the triumph of freedom over servitude. He recognizes that the road to freedom is as difficult as it is rare, but that it is possible to find.

Considering the subtleties of Spinoza's thought, I feel that using it to qualify conscious will as an illusion is a simplification that does not help in understanding the problem of freedom. If free will is only an illusion – as Wegner says – the entire structure of Spinoza's rational thought collapses, and only the psychological study of the sensations that humans experience when they erroneously believe their mind is capable of causing the acts characterizing their conduct makes sense.

The strength of the determinist argument comes from a simple idea: we live in a universe in which all occurrences have a sufficient cause that precedes them. So, if every event is determined by causes that precede it, why would conscious acts be an exception? Traditionally, the idea of "exception" was explained with unscientific, religious, or metaphysical arguments. The point of departure was a fundamental dualism that implied the existence of non-physical, spiritual instances, capable of acting on the physical world. Therefore, the presence of a mysterious agent – the soul – with causal powers over organic matter, was thought to exist. Scientists, most reasonably, reject this argument. However, there is still a problem: the intuition of a large number of people holds the belief that individuals are capable of freely making decisions; and modern civilization has been built on the universally accepted foundation that people are responsible for their acts, to be both rewarded and punished for them. A complex, ramified, and sophisticated set of social, political, and cultural institutions has been constructed as an immense building whose foundation would then be a

---

[21] *Ibid.*, 4th part, proposition 54, note.   [22] *Ibid.*, 4th part, proposition 73.
[23] *Ibid.*, 4th part, appendix, chapter 32.

mere illusion, no doubt useful, but nonetheless a construction elaborated by our brain.

A curious manner of dealing with the problem is to separate two forms of will. The first would be an "empirical will," established by scientific analysis, that is the causal relation between the conscious thoughts of people and the conduct resulting from these. The second would be a "phenomenal will" that is made out of the personal sensations of free will. According to Wegner, the first form of will cannot be directly tied to the second. People mistakenly confuse the sensation of will (phenomenal) with a causal mechanism.[24] However, he admits that the experiences or sensations on which we exercise our will correctly correspond to the real causal connection between thought and action.[25] Of course, he does not clarify whether this "correspondence" has been scientifically proved or if it is only speculative intuition. Nevertheless, if the causal relation between thought and action is contained in a determinist concept, like the one Wegner accepts, then it is totally illogical to speak of an "empirical will" for referring to a causal chain in which freedom is a completely foreign notion. But it is his way of dealing with the reality humans live in; they are not submerged in an incongruous carnival of contingent choices, but rather in societies where many decisions seem to cause actions that correspond to their intentions. Wegner does not want to go as far as Skinner, who totally discarded the notions of responsibility and free will, and so he puts a strange "empirical will" into his interpretation that would have some correlation with the sensations of free will or responsibility and that would be necessary to study as an expression of a type of choice-and-decision phenomenology.

This line of thought leads directly to the conclusion that although freedom is a mere sensation, it is nevertheless a useful illusion. It is advantageous to believe that people should receive rewards and punishments that are guided by an illusory establishment of merits. The sensation of responsibility that is perceived through performing an intentional act is a useful one. Wegner also believes illusion aids in putting the causal puzzle that surrounds us in order. In addition, it can be empirically proved that those who believe in free will are more efficient. When we read his staunch defense that free will is a very useful and comforting illusion, these premises make us end up wondering if it would not be better to opt for silence: why reveal that we are tied to a determinist causal chain if the illusion is so beneficial? According to Wegner, the only advantage to doing away with the illusion is the mental peace that supposedly would overcome us, after resignedly accepting our submission to determinism, instead of dauntlessly fighting for control. This alternative, which is characteristic of Zen Buddhism, proposes to renounce our pretention to intentionally

---

[24] Wegner, *The illusion of conscious will*, pp. 14–15.   [25] *Ibid.*, p. 327.

control the causal chain. But then Wegner realizes that perhaps it is not possible to intentionally renounce the illusion of intentionality. He has fallen into a curious contradiction.[26]

Something similar occurs in quantum physics: Heisenberg explained that the same process of observing the velocity and the position of an electron perturbs it in such a manner that inevitable measuring errors are produced. Likewise, the voluntary act of explaining free will as an illusion inevitably perturbs the study results: if the act effectively is free and conscious, it contradicts the conclusion that free will is an illusion. If the act of studying is subject to a determinist causal chain, nothing guarantees that the conclusion corresponds to reality, because a result showing that free will is a reality and that determinism is an illusion would be equally functional.

Readers may sense that there is something suspiciously wrong in these affirmations. However, many psychologists and neuroscientists reject the idea that consciousness can voluntarily make decisions that produce acts. If consciousness is defined as a process that occurs exclusively within the brain, an almost inevitable mechanical determinist interpretation is arrived at. An idea contrary to this rendering tends to be qualified as metaphysical or Cartesian. Despite everything, I believe that there are clearly materialist and non-metaphysical explanations that enable us to understand that self-consciousness is a process that does not occur totally inside the brain and that it is better understood if we place it in a wider context that includes the social and cultural environment. And we will advance further, especially if we pay attention to what Spinoza said: liberty is based on the *conatus*, the endeavor or the tendency that drives humans to reason and to understand that they are conscious of themselves.

---

[26] In a confusing book on freedom, the philosopher Daniel Dennett is also very contradictory. On the one hand he enthusiastically approves Wegner's basic ideas on free will, but on the other, he disagrees with the exposition tactic of the problem. Dennett believes one must say that freedom is not an illusion and at the same time he approves all the suppositions supporting Wegner. The basic agreement would be in the fact that both believe that moral and responsible actions are real. In other words, he believes in the real effects of the belief in an illusion. Freedom would be like religion: it is false but it produces real beneficial results (*Freedom evolves*, pp. 224–225 and 305). Another more recent book, along the lines of Wegner, puts forth the idea that the "I" is an illusion and falls into the same traps (Hood, *The self illusion*).

16   An experiment with freedom

It is a curious paradox that the neurophysiologist whose experiments are the most widely cited for sustaining determinist theses believed in the existence of free will. Benjamin Libet (1916–2007) was a scientist who became known in the United States in the 1970s for his experiments showing that even when a tactile sensation takes half a second to be consciously reported by the person, it is subjectively perceived as if it had arrived exactly at the same moment. Libet later installed very precise recording instruments in his laboratory for the purpose of measuring the time that passes from the moment a person decides to act (for example, move a finger) and the instant in which it is actually done. He used an electroencephalograph device to record the cerebral cortex activity and an oscilloscope to time the events. It should be mentioned that some ten years before, two German researchers from the University of Freiburg, H. H. Kornhuber and L. Deecke, had discovered what they called *Bereitschaftspotential*, which is the preparation potential that appears in the electroencephalogram moments before a voluntary movement has occurred. Libet's experiment showed that this electric preparation potential happened *before* the subjects manifested their intention to perform an action, but *after* their having consciously decided to do it. He also showed that a voluntary decision could abort the movement, even when the preparation potential had been triggered. More concretely, Libet's experiments indicated that the electric changes that prepare an action in the brain begin some 550 milliseconds *before* the action occurs. The subjects notice the intention to act some 350 to 400 milliseconds *after* the preparation potential begins, but 200 milliseconds *before* the motor action occurs. Libet came to the conclusion that the intentional action began unconsciously. But he also observed that consciousness can control the process result through a kind of vetoing power: it could inhibit the mechanisms that lead to the action, even when they had already begun unconsciously.[1]

---

[1] See Libet's reflections many years after his experiments: "Do we have free will?"

Libet's experiments caused a great commotion. His own conclusions have been severely criticized by the determinists, because he stated that free will was a scientific option that was just as good or better than its denial. He supported his idea through a quote from Isaac Bashevis Singer: "The greatest gift which humanity has received is free choice. It is true that we are limited in our use of free choice. But the little free choice we have is such a great gift and is potentially worth so much that for this itself life is worthwhile living."[2] The determinists praised the result of the experiments that showed that the voluntary act begins unconsciously, but they rejected the possibility that consciousness could interrupt the process. Libet believed that a "conscious mental field" could exist that was capable of acting without neuronal connections functioning as mediators.[3] Certainly he was inspired by the ideas of Karl Popper, who just before his death, defined the mind as a "force field" in one of his reflections presented in 1992.[4] Of course, the problem lies in the supposition of a human activity that has no neuronal support. If this idea is accepted, it opens the door to dualism and non-material mysterious instances capable of moving the body. In this case, we are not very far from imagining the immortal soul moving the body by means of the pineal gland, as Descartes proposed.

In turn, determinism also opened the door to a few demons. For example: if a freely acting will does not exist, then we could have an excuse for any type of immoral behavior because it would always be possible to say that the individual did not commit the offense consciously, but that it came from some uncontrollable mechanical process due to a genetic cause or a biochemical imbalance. An easy way out of this problem is simply to postulate that the moral sense is nothing more than a cerebral device, a set of neuronal circuits mounted in the oldest parts of the primatal brain and configured by natural selection to perform its job, according to Steven Pinker.[5] From this point of view, if the device malfunctions, the cause is not found in the exercise of free will, but in a person's brain module, nevertheless holding the person responsible for her or his acts. In this case the blame does not fall on the soul or on consciousness, but rather on a mechanism that is inserted into a determinist network of cause-and-effect. The guilty party carrying the built-in module equally deserves a punishment or a special (psychiatric) treatment. I will return to these problems further on.

There is an example that seems to indicate that free will is a demonstrable scientific fact. Obsessive-compulsive disorder, which I have already discussed, implies an involuntary intromission of consciousness. One of the most successful ways of combating this disease is the so-called cognitive behavioral therapy. Through its use, people afflicted with this mental disorder have been able to

---

[2] Quoted in *ibid.*, p. 57.   [3] *Ibid.*, p. 56.
[4] Popper, Lindahl and Århem, "A discussion of the mind-brain problem."
[5] Pinker, *The blank slate*, chapter 15.

learn alternate behaviors that substitute the compulsion to, let us say, continually wash their hands. The therapy involves four steps: relabel, reattribute, refocus, and revalue. This means that the patient learns to recognize the intrusive impulse as an effect of the disease, to understand that this is due to a chemical imbalance, to distract his or her attention with an alternative conduct, and to evaluate the symptom in a new way. With this, the psychiatrist Jeffrey Schwartz argues that treatment produces systematic changes in the brain's metabolism of glucose as a result of a series of voluntary decisions carried out by an individual during treatment.

The psychiatrist explains to the patient that the hand-washing urgency comes from an error in the neuronal circuits that sends a false signal, probably produced by an excessive neuronal activity in the networks that connect the caudate nucleus with the orbital and anterior cingulate cortices. Schwartz has demonstrated that cognitive behavioral therapy generates new cerebral circuits thanks to the exercise of will.[6] To explain this situation he turns to the notion of "mental force," similar to the definition of the mind as a "force field" suggested by Popper. This psychiatrist concludes with a hypothesis: that mental force "is a genuine physical force generated by real mental effort."[7] It has also been proved that placebos produce physical effects, which is an added argument to the proposal that a person's mind can exert an influence over his or her body, even though in this case it has been tricked by receiving an innocuous drug substitute.

This argument has not convinced the determinists, who in this example continue to see the camouflaged proposal of a dualist interpretation that accepts that something "mental" (not physical) can exert an influence on the physical machinery of the brain.[8] For them, volition is a mere cerebral action explainable through the determinist mechanisms that the physical sciences postulate and

---

[6] Schwartz, "A role for volition and attention in the generation of new brain circuitry."

[7] *Ibid.*, p. 131. Another example that seems to confirm the power of the conscious will is the system of imaging neurofeedback obtained through functional magnetic resonance (real-time fMRI neurofeedback). The system consists of locating and imaging an area of the brain, modifying the images by computer to transmit them to a screen the person who is being examined can see. The idea is to show a person his or her own brain activity patterns "live" so that he or she can voluntarily modify undesirable or harmful cognitive processes. It has been successfully applied in cases of chronic pain (see Chapin, Bagarinao, and Mackey, "Real-time fMRI applied to pain management"). The system is similar to one that has been used in primates and in tetraplegic people; electrodes are implanted in the brain and the subjects can learn to mentally control a brain-machine connection to move a robotic arm from a distance.

[8] See, for example, Clark, "Fear of mechanism." See another interesting compatibilist interpretation in Díaz, "El cerebro moral, la voluntad y la neuroética," in which he explains that, in the process of decision-making, there is an instant, difficult to determine, in which there is a state of volition and of self-consciousness that must have a still unknown nervous correlation. For him, determinism and free will are compatible: there is a neurophysiological process that has the capacity for self-regulation and direction thanks to its complexity.

that are expressed in neuronal functions. But proceeding from this postulate, the determinists have not been able to add anything toward the comprehension of consciousness, free will, or ethical decisions. It is true that to accept the existence of a "non-physical mind" is a violation of the laws of physics. But to state that the mind has a physical character does not help at all to explain the functioning of the processes that underlie decision-making. It would be like pretending that the physical nature of a social or political institution contributed to the understanding of their functions. The philosopher John Searle has made an effort to explain how there can be types of objective events that only exist due to the fact that we believe in them, such as money, family, taxes, property, or universities. Searle says that these social facts are based on consciousness, language, and rationality, and he further states that all this is the expression of a more fundamental underlying biology.[9] He has also sustained that the different cultures "are different forms that an underlying biological substructure can be manifested in."[10] He is absolutely right in stating that there is no opposition between biology and culture, just as there is also none between body and mind. But he is wrong in concluding that culture is the form biology takes. It seems to me that this is a manifestation of the old reductionism that compresses society into neurons, to then have biology collapse into chemistry, and chemistry into physics.[11]

Admitting the existence of a "mental force" does not help us much either. What kind of force is it? What characteristics does it have? Apparently it is an interaction that has nothing to do with Newtonian or quantum mechanics, nor does it seem to be understood in relation to the molecular mechanics studied by chemists. Moreover, we can understand that the behavior of neurons can hardly be qualified as "free" or "determined," just as it makes no sense to assert that individual particles are solid, liquid, or gas. These states are properties of the set of particles. The free or determined state only makes sense in the system or set formed by the brain and its surroundings. Whether determination and freedom can coexist in the set is what needs to be studied, but while doing so we must not fall into the Cartesian dualism and find ourselves forced to tie free will together with the presence of mysterious metaphysical forces (or physical ones of an indefinite nature).

Freedom cannot be understood if consciousness is locked inside the brain. When many neuroscientists insist on rejecting this idea, they condemn their research and reflection to remaining trapped in a vicious circle, in which free will is nothing more than an illusion created by the brain, a mere epiphenomenon

---

[9] Searle, *Freedom and neurobiology*, p. 12. See a sharp criticism of the reductionism of Searle in Hofstadter, *I am a strange loop*, pp. 28–31.
[10] Searle, *The construction of social reality*, p. 227.
[11] See a critique of this reductionism in Rose, *Lifelines*.

that is perhaps necessary or useful, but that lacks causal power. This idea leaves us with no explanation of free will, which can then only be seen as a political expression possessing an enormous philosophical and literary aura, but that would be nothing more than a link in a determinist chain housed in the human brain. If, in contrast, we broaden our perspective and understand consciousness as a set of cerebral and exocerebral networks, we can discover facets and processes that a narrow vision is unable to comprehend.

I would like to outline some aspects that can be discovered precisely if we broaden our perspective. First, as Spinoza had already suspected, it must be recognized that free will is a scarce good. What I mean is that not all human acts are the result of freedom: only a small part of human activity escapes the deterministic mechanisms. The important thing here is to emphasize that *yes*, free acts are possible and that a fraction of what we do forms part of a social space in which conscious will is an important causal element. This conscious will cannot be reduced to a neuronal (or molecular) scale or to the level of small acts (like moving a finger) that some neuroscientists have studied. We can only understand it as part of a system, at the level of social and cultural interactions, in which of course the neuronal networks of the involved individuals intervene. Conscious will would be a property or a condition of a system of cerebral and exocerebral networks. And finally, to finish this sketch, I wish to state that the process of choosing freely and consciously is not an instantaneous one: it can last hours and days. If we decompensate it in a series of instantaneous micro-decisions, we will lose the image of the set. In the case of experiments such as those of Libet, we can understand that the decision to move actually began at the moment the study subjects agreed to voluntarily participate in the tests.[12] The philosopher Shaun Gallagher has rightly stated: "Freely willed action is some-thing accomplished in the world, in situations that motivate embedded reflec-tion, and amongst the things that I reach for and the people that I affect."[13]

Therefore, it is necessary to place the problem of free will at a higher level of complexity, and by doing so, not to forget that there are underlying neuronal, chemical, and physical structures. Certainly, elevating the level of complexity by introducing the social and cultural structures does not resolve the problem: it places it in a context in which it is possible to carry out more productive research. But it must be recognized that things apparently become complicated, because by accepting that consciousness is also an exocerebral phenomenon, new variables are introduced, the most important of which is the network of

---

[12] See Deecke and Kornhuber, "Human freedom, reasoned will, and the brain"; Mele, "Decision, intentions, urges, and free will."

[13] Gallagher, "Where's the action?" p. 123. This author maintains that Libet's experiments do not show if we have free will or not because this concept does not apply to movements studied in the laboratory.

symbolic processes, without which conscious will cannot exist. The problem becomes tangled for those who wish to approach the theme of consciousness strictly through the discipline of neurology, and who mistakenly assume that the introduction of exocerebral variables is like opening the door to metaphysics. The network of exocerebral symbolic processes is not a metaphysical phenomenon, but rather a solid reality rooted in the materiality of the world, and it cannot be reduced to biochemical and physical explanations. The study of the interaction between the neuronal and symbolic networks places us in front of a more complex situation, but one that can facilitate – not complicate – the understanding of the mental mechanisms of free will.

I want to give an example of what it can mean to reduce will to brain mechanisms. The neurologist Mark Hallett maintains that free will is not a force that determines movement.[14] The process that triggers movements, according to Hallett, occurs subconsciously and the sensation of will arises after the movement is begun. Hallett concludes that movement is probably initiated in the middle motor area under the influence of the prefrontal and limbic areas of the brain. The order to move goes to the primary motor cortex and culminates in discharges in the parietal area. This last area maintains relatively constant bilateral connections with the frontal area and it is likely that the insula also intervenes. The perception that movement is the result of will is generated within this neuronal network. And so it is the motor mechanisms of the brain that generate the sensation that there are free decisions that cause the movement. In conclusion, the question arises as to whether people are responsible for their behavior if free will is not the motor force of movement. It appears to be a difficult problem, but actually it is not. The solution is simple: "A person's brain is clearly fully responsible, and always responsible, for the person's behavior." Hallett believes behavior is a product of a person's experience and genes. The mechanisms that cause movement, house experiences, perceive sensations, generate emotions, and produce homeostatic impulses function in the neuronal circuitry. No free will exists there.

So, yes, there is an innocent or guilty party responsible for our actions: the brain. This neurologist comes to a symptomatic conclusion: a person's behavior is influenced by external interventions, such as reward and punishment. He recognizes that there are social decisions that can correct the behavior emanating from people's brains (whose will power is nothing more than a perception). If we follow the logic of his argument, we would be facing an almost infinite

[14] Hallett, "Volitional control of movement." David Eagleman, a neuroscientist with a wide-ranging readership, has published similar ideas. He believes that the studies of the brain have ousted us from the place we thought we occupied in the center of ourselves; consciousness has been dethroned, but far from seeming depressing, this appears magical to him. There is no conscious mind that steers the ship or any test that demonstrates the existence of free will, according to Eagleman (*Incognito*, pp. 169, 193, 224).

regression: the prizes and punishments would simply be the apparently free decisions of a multitude of associated brains, responding to the determinations of the neuronal networks of each one.

We are not obligated to follow behaviorist logic. We can explore other paths, such as those I have mentioned that lead us to examine the relation between the neuronal networks and the sociocultural environment. The example that I have just briefly explored – of punishments and rewards – takes us directly to the question of morality, the theme of the next chapter.

17   The moral brain

People are continuously faced with the need to make moral decisions and to act upon them accordingly. Some psychologists sustain the idea that there is an inborn cerebral module in humans that is responsible for the unconscious and automatic process that produces judgments about right and wrong. This idea is a transfer of the postulates of Noam Chomsky on the existence of a generative grammar housed in the neuronal circuitry, to the field of ethics.[1] Likewise, there would be a moral grammar, a kind of instinct dwelling in the brain that, from unconscious and inaccessible principles, would generate judgments on what is permissible, prohibited, unjust, and correct. Of course a moral instinct (or faculty) would generate different rules and customs in each cultural context, in the same way that the brain module of language is supposed to produce different languages in individuals in accordance with where they are born and raised. But the module would impose the same grammatical structure in all cases.

A book by Marc Hauser, a professor of psychology at Harvard University, has popularized this interpretation.[2] He maintains that the moral instinct has been developed throughout the process of evolution and is more apparent in the intuition of humans than in their reasoning. These instincts color our perceptions and restrict moral judgments. However, Hauser does not explicitly indicate what the universal moral principles that are lodged in the moral organ of our brain are, perhaps because he believes that these principles, "tucked away in the mind's library of unconscious knowledge, are inaccessible."[3] But at one point he exemplifies what would be a universal principle. Infanticide, he says, is regarded as a barbaric act in the United States. In contrast, among the Eskimos – and in other cultures – infanticide is morally permissible and justifiable in view of the great scarcity of resources. It would seem that there are opposing moral

---

[1] The philosopher Hilary Putnam rightly ironizes the ideas of Chomsky: "To say that 'the universal grammar in the brain' generates the 'semantic component' when the values of certain parameters have been 'properly set by the environment' is to say that we-know-not-what does we-know-not-what when we-know-not-what has happened!" (*The threefold cord*, p. 124.)
[2] Hauser, *Moral minds*.   [3] *Ibid.*, p. 2.

principles here. But Hauser explains that, in reality, the Eskimos as well as Americans are guided by the same universal principle: the obligation to take care of children. What varies in the different cultures are the *exceptions* to the rule. His conclusion is simple: "our moral faculty is equipped with a set of universal rules, and each culture establishes particular exceptions to these rules."[4] I have my doubts that caring for children is a moral principle. If it were, then the search for food or the fleeing from dangerous predators would also have to be considered moral principles that not only are universal among humans, but also are shared with a vast number of animals. In other passages of the book, he mentions certain prohibitions, such as injustice, unfaithfulness, incest, murder, and the infliction of pain, but it is not clear if he regards them as universal principles that could give rise to exceptions in the different cultures. Hauser's general argument establishes that morality is based on or rooted in biology. Therefore, he maintains that we are provided with a universal moral grammar, which means that "general but abstract principles for deciding which actions are prohibited, permissible, or obligatory" have evolved within us and that "these principles lack specific content."[5] The innate abstract principles do not dictate to us which acts are permissible, unless culture and education provide them with content and decide what the exceptions are. Apparently, the moral module would not flow directly into the individuals, but only when mediated by culture. But the book is full of examples of individual "intuitions" that seemingly would be caused by the functioning of the innate moral faculty. The obligation to take care of children (supposing that it is a moral rule) is an imperative for which there can certainly be exceptions. The same holds true for the principles prohibiting killing or stealing. Let us look at an example used by Hauser. Like most of his examples, it is an imaginary situation (and a bit absurd). In a modern western nation any person would feel offended if a buyer offered a thousand dollars for each of his or her children. What would that person think if the offer were a million dollars? What would the reaction be if it were a billion dollars or some other exorbitant amount? Those who would succumb to the temptation would feel very guilty. Hauser asks: what is it in such a situation that offends us? If we asked people they would not know how to explain it; there are simply taboos prohibiting certain things from entering into the market. I do not agree: people would surely give many explanations as to why the buying and selling of human beings and slavery are prohibited. Every

---

[4] *Ibid.*, p. 44. In relation to the cultural variations of morality, see the suggestive and much more sophisticated reflections of the anthropologist James Faubion on the multiple subject positions from which the conscious practice of freedom is exercised; in his book *An Anthropology of Ethics* he shows that ethical variability places ethics in the realm of intersubjective phenomena. His starting point is Michel Foucault's assertion that the freedom of the subject and its relations to others is the very stuff of ethics.

[5] Hauser, *Moral minds*, p. 420.

culture, asserts Hauser, "has the freedom to decide which items enter into legitimate business and which are off limits." And he adds: "Continuing with the linguistic analogy, I would say that every culture has a fairness principle in reference to exchanges, with a parameter that the local culture establishes for what is exchangeable."[6] The problem is that people do not have access to the underlying principles that generate judgments and so they respond to the prohibitions as if they were taboos. But the astute psychologist *does* know that there are underlying principles, which enables him to consciously think about something that – at any rate – is already contained in the moral module of his own brain. What is *not* clear is how the psychologist knows that justice is recorded in his neuronal networks, and that this, in reality, is not the result of his having read the works of John Rawls.

It is supposed that the moral faculty inserted in the brain is a product of evolution. This affirmation is connected to David Hume's famous determinist thesis, which holds that reason is the slave of the passions and cannot do anything but serve and obey them. This means that the moral sense is analogous to the physical senses, which are the product of biological evolution. But Hauser moves away from Hume's thesis in order to defend the moral principles of the Enlightenment tradition handed down from Kant and embodied in Rawls. His model is a curious mixture of Rawls and Chomsky, in which he grafts the inborn moral faculty onto the rational process of analyzing causes and consequences. The amalgam of rational analysis with the innate module of moral principles comes from the comparison that Rawls himself made between the formation of the sense of justice and the sense of grammaticality studied by Chomsky (through which we recognize well-formed phrases in our language).[7] Nevertheless, the fusion of Rawls with the determinist modular interpretations is something that is completely forced and can only be explained by the intention of introducing liberal ethics into a schema that he obviously is not comfortable with.

Steven Pinker, the inspiration for Hauser's thesis, did something similar.[8] The moral sense would be a product of reciprocal altruism inserted in a natural evolutionary process, whose expansion would be stimulated through personal interactions and cultural exchange among people. These factors would have caused a broadening of the networks of reciprocity that ended in the respect for other humans seen as beings more valuable alive than dead, which supposedly would be contained in the moral module. Pinker came to the following

---

[6] *Ibid.*, p. 158.

[7] Rawls, *A theory of justice*, p. 47. See a good critique of Hauser's ideas in Churchland, *Braintrust*, pp. 104ff. There is political motivation in Chomsky's insistence on declaring the existence of inborn mental structures; in an interview in 1969 he said that if there were none, there would be those who would want to control that plasticity or that randomness to mold behavior by means of State authority, behaviorist technology, or some other medium ("Linguistics and politics").

[8] Pinker, *The blank slate*.

conclusion: "The moral sense is a gadget, like stereo vision or intuitions about number. It is an assembly of neural circuits cobbled together from older parts of the primate brain and shaped by natural selection to do a job."[9] Naturally, there is no scientific proof that these moral modules exist. The geneticist H. Allen Orr regards Pinker's proposal as ridiculous:

The notion that our moral circle expanded by reciprocity is in many cases ahistorical nonsense. Men had plenty of "people-to-people" interaction with women while condemning them to second-class citizenship. And slaveholding Southerners had more "cultural exchanges" and "people-to-people activities" with African-Americans than did abolitionist Northerners. At what point in history did our "networks of reciprocity" with women and slaves become sufficiently dense that the calculus of reciprocity demanded that we grant them the vote and freedom? The question is absurd.[10]

Pinker, in a reply, accepted that in addition to the mechanisms of reciprocity, "universalist sensibility" and the "constraints of rational argumentation" should have been taken into account.[11]

I have cited the arguments of Hauser and Pinker to demonstrate a different facet of the question of free will. For them, decisions are inscribed in the functioning of an innate moral module that is a type of neurological program performing specific tasks. We can see how this explanation is greatly influenced by computer science and cybernetics. The mechanisms of the module restrict the degrees of freedom of the individuals faced with the task of decision-making in the presence of moral dilemmas. I would like to give another example of this type of explanation, even though in this case the model refers to the way in which the brain recognizes and internalizes moral virtues. Paul Churchland designed a theory about how moral knowledge functions. According to him, the neuronal network incorporates abilities when it receives moral information. Discernment capacity resides in an intricate matrix of synaptic connections that houses categories and subcategories that refer to specific situations such as "lies," "betrayal," "theft," "torture," "murder," and so on. There is an acquired set of moral prototypes that forms a structure, a kind of map that lets us effectively navigate through a social world that is constantly demanding ethical decisions.[12] Everything takes place in the biological *hardware* of the

---

[9] *Ibid.*, p. 270. This book, after defending the obvious idea that there is no original blank slate, sets forth the Chomskyan idea about the presence of modules in the brain. The existence of inherited capacities can be proven, for example, in what Stanislas Dehaene called the "number sense," a capacity to rapidly perceive the approximate number of objects, which is shared with some animals (see his book *The number sense*). The idea of innate moral tendencies inscribed in the brain has been carried to the extreme of supposing, for example, six basic modules, each one responsible for a duality of values: care/harm, liberty/oppression, fairness/cheating, loyalty/ betrayal, authority/subversion, and sanctity/degradation (Haidt, *The righteous mind*).
[10] Orr, "Darwinian storytelling," p. 20.
[11] Pinker and Orr, "*The blank slate*: an exchange," p. 48.
[12] Churchland, "Toward a cognitive neurobiology of moral virtues."

brain, which Churchland defines as a massive parallel vectorial processor. This image largely comes from connectionist studies conducted on artificial intelligence models. Only neurobiological research will be able to prove or disprove this explanation.[13] What I wish to underline here is that there is no assumption of the existence of inborn rules contained in modules. On the contrary, moral experience goes along building a great diversity of prototypes; these prototypes encode the acquired knowledge at points in the neuronal space, each one possessing as many dimensions and characteristics as possible. No rules or moral principles can be fixed onto these neuronal vectors: what exists is a multitude of prototypes.

This model suffers from the same defect the theory of inborn modules does: it does not take the structure and peculiarities of the external flow of moral information into consideration. The language here is a system that translates social experiences into another internal language, which could be called a kind of Neuralese, with which the gigantic vectorial processor that encodes ethical prototypes operates. The defect, as pointed out by Andy Clark, is in the fact that language is also a complement that increases the computational power of the brain through signs, words, and labels. Clark said that public language is a reservoir of useful re-codings that have accumulated in a slow and painful cultural process of trial and error, and that it reduces patterns that are too complex and are cognitively invisible to regular and recognizable ones that enable the brain to carry out a sharper exploration of the moral space. Inspired in the ideas of the linguist Lev Vygotsky, Clark referred to all of this as the "external scaffolding" of human cognition.[14] Paul Churchland took this criticism well and accepted the notion that part of the cognitive machinery is situated outside the brain, in the discursive scaffolding that structures the social world and that is made up of drawn diagrams, written arithmetic calculations, spoken and printed arguments, tools of measurement and manipulation, and cognitive prostheses.[15] But the scaffolds are provisional support structures that are dismantled and removed, once the objective has been achieved. The metaphor of a prosthesis, or even better, a permanent exocerebrum, without which the neuronal networks of humans cannot function correctly, is much more useful.

Whether the brain is seen as a vectorial processor that internalizes moral information flows with the help of social scaffolding or is considered to house

[13] There is an interesting application of the computer model to the processes of consciousness made by Daniel Bor. This neuroscientist says it is possible that in the future an artificial consciousness will be developed. For Bor the brain is a kind of computer that functions very similarly to its first cousins, the electronic machines that process information, and therefore it is logical for them to develop forms of consciousness similar to humans (*The Ravenous Brain*).

[14] Clark, "Word and action."

[15] Churchland, "Rules, know-how, and the future of moral cognition."

innate modules that are responsible for the generative flow that reaches society, the moral operations in both cases are located in the neuronal networks. The difference between them is that in the first case, the innate computational machinery assimilates external rules in the form of prototypes, and in the second, the modules contain innate generative principles. The fact that the decision-making process does not take place exclusively inside the head, but occurs in permanent relation between the brain and its sociocultural environment, escapes both interpretations. The environment is not just the source that nurtures the learning process, nor is it the receptor context that adapts the generative flows of the neuronal modules. A substantial part of this environment is permanently connected to the neuronal network, in the same way that the biologist Jakob von Uexküll defined the *Umwelt*, the subjective universe of an organism, where each component has a functional significance for him. It operates with a set of receptor and effector signs that link the organism to its own *Umwelt*.[16] The anthropologist Gregory Bateson, in his reflections on what he called an "ecology of mind," also understood that consciousness is part of a broad system that includes the social and the natural environments that surround the individual. His thoughts are very stimulating, but they are also excessively conditioned by a cybernetic concept of the processes linking the "I" with the outside world. Bateson places consciousness in a homeostatic and cybernetic system. He recognizes that consciousness can be a causal element that feeds back into the networks of the self-regulated system that it forms part of. He suggests that the true cybernetic nature of the "I" and of the world tends not to be perceived by consciousness. We are blind and do not see the cybernetic circularity of the "I" and the world. Nevertheless, the cybernetic interpretations of the mental and brain processes, so popular a few decades ago, do not culminate in very illuminating results.[17]

We must open a new door to understand the question of free will. There are decisions that are made in the hybrid circuits of consciousness that include the brain and the exocerebrum in the same network; there is a space here for free will, and not because the door to chance or chaos is opened, now that the exocerebrum is embedded in a very well-structured social and cultural world. What needs to be explored is whether the confluence of different factors, those

---

[16] Uexküll, "A stroll through the worlds of animals and men." See also how Ernst Cassirer bases his idea of man as a symbolic animal on Uexküll *(An Essay on Man*, chapter 2).

[17] Bateson, *Steps to an ecology of mind*, especially the essay "Effects of conscious purpose on human adaptations" (1968). A more general theoretical proposition concerning the links that connect the brain with the cultural spaces has been suggested by the anthropologist Stephen P. Reyna in his book *Connections*. Reyna proposes the existence of an internal "neurohermeneutic system" – a "connector" – that would receive information from the exterior through sensory receptors, process it, produce neuronal signals, and send a response to the cultural spaces. Just like the proposals regarding the existence of translating apparatuses or modules inside the brain, the idea of an internal neurohermeneutic system lacks demonstrable support.

that originate in the nervous system and those that come from the world that surrounds us, allows for a process of free choice. The easy way to escape the determinism that understands freedom as an illusion is simply to deny the influence of biological factors on decisions, in order to postulate that it is the social, cultural, and political instances that, in any case, decide if there is freedom or not. Here, too, we would fluctuate between determinist and libertarian theses, but the parameters of the discussion would remain restricted (and reduced) to the social processes. "Human nature" and biology would not have the right to take the floor.

But we would not get very far in this flight that is typical of those who are afraid to confront the unavoidable fact of our biological reality. We have no choice but to try to understand the mystery of free will from the intimate connection between our biological constitution and social life, between the brain and culture.

18   Unchained reasons

There is a forceful statement by the great Scottish philosopher David Hume that is often cited by the determinists: "Reason is and ought only to be the slave of the passions."[1] Hume, in his *Treatise* of 1740, rejects a theory of freedom that does not accept the basic principles of causality and necessity, because he believes that if they are removed then freedom is eliminated by chance. In this context he establishes that reason cannot cause any action on its own, because for this to happen, it must be accompanied by the passions. Eight years later in *An Enquiry Concerning Human Understanding* (1748), he once again insisted on the determinist theme: "It is universally allowed that nothing exists without a cause of its existence, and that chance, when strictly examined, is a mere negative word, and means not any real power which has anywhere a being in nature." And a bit further on he explains that freedom, when opposed to necessity, is identical to chance, which does not exist, because Hume understands chance as a situation that is not produced by any cause.[2] However, in this scientific and empiricist context, Hume left us a definition of liberty: "By liberty, then, we can only mean a power of acting or not acting, according to the determinations of the will; this is, if we choose to remain at rest, we may; if we choose to move, we also may." This freedom – which is not chance – is universally accepted as belonging to all those who are neither prisoners, nor in chains.[3]

In his *Treatise*, Hume had already used the dismal example of a prisoner to show the interrelation between voluntary acts and natural causes. He refers to a prisoner condemned to death who has no money or help, and who discovers that it is impossible to escape: he is trapped in a causal chain that includes both the will of his jailors, as well as the iron bars and stone walls that hold him captive. When the prisoner arrives at the scaffold he can unmistakably foresee his death and his mind runs through the causal chain: "The refusal of the soldiers to consent to his escape, the action of the executioner; the separation of the head

---

[1] Hume, *A Treatise of Human Nature*, book II, part III, section III.
[2] Hume, *An Enquiry Concerning Human Understanding*, section VIII, part I, § 74.
[3] *Ibid.*, section VIII, part I, § 73.

and body; bleeding, convulsive motions." This macabre description aids Hume in concluding that there is "a connected chain of natural causes and voluntary actions; but the mind feels no difference betwixt them in passing from one link to another."[4] The iron of the bars is as inflexible as the will of the jailors. The physical causes in the causal chain have the same effect as the volitive acts. Nevertheless, Hume realized that the freedom to act can change the course of a process, but not because that freedom was located outside the enchainment of causes and effects. In contrast, if freedom is understood as an example of "determinations of the will," that is precisely what makes it possible to define the responsibility of the punishable or rewardable acts of humans. An act that is the product of pure chance, whether malignant or benign, does not let us attribute merit or penalty to its producer. Hume accepts the compatibility of liberty and necessity, even though his explanation is more utilitarian than scientific. Liberty is the capacity to decide *within* a cause-and-effect network. Outside of this network, liberty is chance, and does not exist.

Unlike Spinoza, for whom the free individual is one that lives only by the dictates of reason, Hume is convinced that reason alone can never be the cause of an action. Morality cannot be based only on reason, which is inert; the passions are required to propel moral actions. It should be pointed out that Hume uses a precise and narrow definition of reason: it is the discovery of what is true and what is false; but reason is incapable of determining good and bad. Here is not the place to discuss the subtleties of Hume's theory in relation to the passions. I only wish to return to the example of the series of causes and effects that shackle the prisoner that is condemned to death. Let us suppose that one of his jailors, out of a pious or generous passion, decided to let him escape during the night. Here is the intervention of a voluntary action, motivated by a passion, and perhaps together with a reason, that modifies the causal chain imagined by Hume that would necessarily lead to the scaffold. The Scottish philosopher foresaw this possibility when he accepted the existence of a form of liberty, but he did not explore its consequences.

If we observe the list of passions that Hume presents, we can notice that many of them are similar to what Antonio Damasio has called "social emotions."[5] If we follow Hume's argument on pride and humility, two passions that he dedicates many pages to, it does not take long to realize that they are part of a peculiar relation between the self and its surrounding society. He even goes as far as saying that property, together with its accompanying wealth, is what stimulates pride the most. For Hume, property is a particular type of causation and he has no doubt in maintaining that it bestows *liberty* upon the owner: a liberty to do what he or she will with that possession and to enjoy the benefits

[4] Hume, *A Treatise of Human Nature*, book II, part III, section I.
[5] Damasio, *The feeling of what happens*, pp. 50–51.

gained from it.[6] But I am interested in emphasizing the fact that many of the passions that Hume calls indirect (such as vanity, hatred, generosity, ambition, and piety, in addition to pride and humility) are clearly social emotions, even though they are doubtlessly linked to what he calls the "direct" passions that are produced by pain or pleasure, by evil or by good. Damasio adds jealousy, embarrassment, and guilt, to which we could include regret, shame, indignation, and disdain. These social emotions occur in the hybrid circuits of consciousness, in the networks that join the brain with the exocerebrum.

With this brief excursion through the ideas of Hume, I have wanted to show that it is unnecessary, even from the perspective of the great importance of the emotions in moral life, to put forward the determinist idea of there being a moral sense similar to the physical senses. Contrary to what some people think, Hume did not believe in that postulate. For him, the sense of justice is artificial, rather than natural, and has its origin in education and a series of conventions that are established for regulating, for example, property rights.[7]

So now we can understand that education and the established social institutions are not mere constructions made from emotional impulses and the desires they provoke. Correlations of strength, negotiations, pacts, and a certain accumulation of rational thoughts and deliberations crystallize into the established conventions. Passion does not always rule and reason is not invariably its slave in the social space of the established conventions. The social space cannot be reduced to a series of emotions and reasons. In society there are traditions, structures, symbols, myths, customs, riches, diseases, beliefs, and systems, to name a few elements whose natures and interactions cannot be the emotional or rational substrate of individuals. However, the possibility of a free exercise of will crystallizes into individual decisions and acts, even though they are mediated by society. Here is where great care must be taken to avoid a pitfall: by escaping from physical determinism we could stay trapped in social determinism.

Society is made up of individuals provided with consciousness and this consciousness has causal powers. These powers that obviously rely on the emotions, propel individuals to make decisions based on reflection and deliberation. This deliberation can be rational, as Spinoza wanted. But it can also be irrational – in other words, based on a deliberate series of reflections that we cannot consider rational because they harm society, other individuals, and sometimes, the same person making the decisions. What is interesting to point out here is the existence

---

[6] Hume, *A Treatise of Human Nature*, book II, part I, section X, "Of property and riches": "If justice, therefore, be a virtue, which has a natural and original influence on the human mind, property may be look'd upon as a particular species of causation; whether we consider the liberty it gives the proprietor to operate as he please upon the object or the advantages, which he reaps from it."

[7] *Ibid.*, book III, part II, section I, "Justice, whether a natural or artificial virtue?"

of voluntary acts that are not completely *determined* by sufficient previous causes, even though they are *influenced* by them. Here consciousness is the original cause in the process itself, or as was expressed in the past; it is *natura naturans* and not *natura naturata*. This situation involves the coexistence of indeterminism and deliberation, something very similar to Spinoza's *conatus*. But this indetermination does not indicate a behavior that is subject to mere chance; it is possible because consciousness is an articulation between the brain and society. What I like to call singularity occurs in this confluence – that is, a situation in which humans can carry out acts that are not determined, but neither are they random. It is a type of behavior that is not subject to chance and in which it is not possible to define a causal determination. I am not proposing the transfer of notions of mathematics and physics onto the terrain of conscious and voluntary functions. Free will is not, nor is it like, a black hole – that gravitational singularity that physicists study. What I wish to indicate through the idea of singularity is the fact that, in the articulation between the brain and human society, an artificial situation is produced that cannot be reduced to the causal explanations characteristic of biology and physics. Freedom is something rare in nature and it is found only in humans (and perhaps in some higher mammals in a very embryonic form).

It can be very appealing at times to resort to physics in an attempt to explain the singular phenomenon of free will. The philosopher John Searle understands that the experience of freedom simultaneously contains indeterminism and deliberation (or rationality). And when he looks for some form of indeterminism in nature he finds it – as Tagore had done much earlier – in quantum physics. His hypothesis is that consciousness is a manifestation of quantum indeterminism. However, he recognizes that this is not the solution to the problem of free will: he has simply transferred the problem to the level of quantum physics.[8] But this reduction does not seem to be capable of clearing up the mystery.

There are other forms of reductionism that are not concerned with exploring the extensions of the brain into society and culture, either. One of these interpretations reduces consciousness, not to the level of neuronal networks or even to that of quantum physics, but to the realm of information. The advantage of this reduction would be that, thanks to modern information theories, consciousness

---

[8] Searle, *Freedom and neurobiology*, pp. 74ff. Henric Walter has offered a sophisticated "compatibilist" way out to explain the coexistence of free will and determinism. In essence Walter does not believe in free will and posits the alternative idea of "natural autonomy." He rejects the existence of a special causality that would characterize the action of free causal agents. He regards the last links in the causal chain in which humans that consider themselves free intervene as recursive "loops" of volition in which there is an "emotional identification" (Walter, *Neurophilosophy of free will*). Kristin Andrews, in a critique of this book, states that Walter offers us a theory of error, rather than a theory of free will, that explains why we feel that we are free. In fact, Walter explains that humans can have something different in situations that are *similar* to those in which they have acted, but they cannot have something different under *identical* conditions. And so they make the mistake of believing they are free (Andrews, "Review of *Neurophilosophy of free will*").

could be quantitatively represented. In this manner, symbols, concepts, metaphors, ironies, conventions, values, beliefs, and institutions escape from the social and cultural space; they can all be reduced to information.

According to these theories, which are a curious variety of panpsychism, there is consciousness not only in brains, but also in every artifact or system that functions by means of integrated information, whether it be a computer, a smartphone, a thermostat, or a photodiode. It is not about extensions of human consciousness outside the brain. In accordance with this interpretation, as expressed by Giulio Tononi, "at the fundamental level, consciousness is integrated information."[9] His idea is to translate the quantity and quality of the information generated by an integrated system into the language of mathematics and geometry. This theory states that "consciousness depends exclusively on the ability of a system to generate integrated information."[10] As such, consciousness is graded; that is to say, there is a continuum that can extend from a binary photodiode (which has exactly one bit of consciousness) up to the mammalian cerebral cortex, which is endowed with an immensely large quantity of consciousness. According to this theory, which is diametrically opposed to my hypothesis regarding the exocerebrum, consciousness is an intrinsic property: in other words, "a complex generating integrated information is conscious in a certain way regardless of any extrinsic perspective."[11] He thus concludes that if consciousness is intrinsic, it is also solipsistic, and that "it could exist in and of itself, without requiring anything extrinsic to it, not even a function or purpose . . . Such a system would not even need any contact with the external world, and it could be completely passive, watching its own states change without having to act."[12]

This proposal has been taken up by Christof Koch, who previously had argued with Francis Crick that consciousness could be explained by the synchronized firing of neurons. He now believes that subjectivity "is too radically different from anything physical for it to be an emergent phenomenon."[13] Because the mental and the physical are two properties that do not permit the one to be reduced into the other, it must be postulated that both are joined together by the mathematics of

[9] Tononi, "Consciousness as integrated information," p. 217.   [10] *Ibid.*, p. 232.
[11] *Ibid.*, p. 233.
[12] *Ibid.*, p. 239. He believes that some day it could be possible "to construct a highly conscious solipsistic entity" (pp. 239–240). In contrast, the anthropologist Clifford Geertz understood that thought is a construct and manipulation of symbolic systems that are used as models of other systems, a perspective that is characteristic of the so-called "extrinsic theory." Thought "consists not of ghostly happenings in the head but of a matching of the states and processes of symbolic models against the states and processes of the wider world." Geertz, *The interpretation of cultures*, p. 214. The "extrinsic theory" was developed in 1956 by the psychologist Eugene Galanter and the mathematician Murray Gerstenhaber ("On thought").
[13] Koch, *Consciousness*, p. 118.

integrated information developed by Giulio Tononi. There is no reduction to the physical here: there is a Pythagorean reduction of the mental to information. Ideas, emotions, or memories can indeed be translated into numbers, actually into binary signals (bits). The same thing that is lost when consciousness is said to be the synchronization of neuronal firing is lost with this reduction as well, despite the fact that it can be extended to non-biological systems. Koch is also convinced that self-consciousness is not concerned with the external world, but rather is directed at interior states,[14] thereby blocking all possibility of comprehending human consciousness that, in my view, is not understandable without its external symbolic networks. This hybrid character of human consciousness cannot be explained by the information theory. Obviously, Koch rejects the possibility of free will, even though he accepts the fact that the old determinism is no longer valid, since quantum mechanics has paved the way for chance.

From my perspective, the mathematics of information works with a flow of signals, not symbols. I use the distinction that Susanne Langer makes of both concepts, which I have already mentioned in chapter 9. Consciousness, among other things, is a translation of signals to symbols, whereas the mathematics of information translates symbols back into signs; however, it is more a reduction than a translation, because it pushes the content itself aside, placing the emphasis on its encoding and transmission. This results in a codification that reduces symbols to signals (bits).

I believe, however, that it is much more productive to go in the opposite direction, not toward physics or mathematics, but toward social and cultural structures. Consciousness and free will do not have a physical or mathematical explanation. We can only understand them if we study the networks that join the brain circuitry with the sociocultural fabrics. That is where we find what I have called the exocerebrum. The study of this set of prostheses that makes up the exocerebrum leads us directly to artifices that are closely linked to the theme of freedom. Artistic, literary, and musical expressions – which are based on symbolic communication structures – can be regarded as the forms through which consciousness is capable of freely expressing itself and of making decisions that trigger causal processes of great creativity that are both innovating and irreducible to determinist explanations. The exocerebrum is a symbolic system that substitutes the cerebral circuits that are incapable by themselves of completing functions that are characteristic of human mental behavior. The brain is not capable of processing symbols without the help of an external system essentially made up of speech, the non-discursive forms of communication (such as music, dance, and painting), and the exterior artificial memories (from writing to the Internet). In the first part of this book, I explored the peculiarities of these basic

---

[14] *Ibid.*, p. 38.

elements of the exocerebrum. Underlying this examination, of course, is the idea that consciousness is a causal agent that can exercise free will. Now I wish to broaden the exploration to other exocerebral expressions, which will allow me to discuss the problem of freedom, of free will as the expression of a consciousness that is not shackled to a despotic determinist chain.

19   Freedom in play

Play is one of the human activities that has most often been associated with freedom. When humans play, they are in that peculiar space where their activities do not seem to be necessary or useful, and where free will rules. The best studies on play have not ceased to point out that it is a free and apparently superfluous behavior. Johan Huizinga, in his extraordinary book, *Homo ludens*, states that one of the main characteristics of play is that it is free.[1] Jean Piaget, the great psychologist, says that play "is the free activity *par excellence*"; he thinks that children's play is accompanied by a feeling of freedom and that it announces art, which is the expansion and flourishing of this spontaneous activity.[2] And Roger Caillois, in his brilliant reflection on play, establishes freedom as its first characteristic.[3]

Play is a free and voluntary activity that at the same time involves a regulated order. This combination places play on the same plane as other exocerebral expressions such as music, dance, and the visual arts. All forms of play follow rules and at the same time are the result of free voluntary decisions in which it is difficult to see an immediate function or usefulness. Games of competition establish rules to ensure equal opportunities and to direct the development of the confrontation, whether they are in sports (soccer, racing, track and field) or of an intellectual nature (chess, go, checkers). In simulation games, in which the participants play the role of a character, an object, or an animal, the conditions and regulations are more flexible, but nevertheless they are indispensable for the ludic exercise. In the cases of mock battle, rules even exist when the players are animals; for example, puppies and kittens engage with one another, but do not hurt each other because they control the force of their biting and swiping. Children that play at being pirates, cowboys, Indians, police officers, thieves, soldiers, astronauts, or firefighters follow certain unwritten rules and place limits on the representation. Games of chance develop according to previously agreed-upon norms and principles. Also, games that are strictly motor exercises

---

[1] Huizinga, *Homo ludens*, p. 20.
[2] Piaget, *La formation du symbole chez l'enfant*, pp. 143, 159.
[3] Caillois, *Les jeux et les hommes*, p. 42.

such as jumping, spinning, rolling about, or running around in circles involve
the following of patterns and rhythms that guide the repetition with variations of
the movements.[4]

Roger Caillois has correctly asserted that rules are inseparable from play the
instant it acquires an institutional existence. However, he says, "a basic freedom
is central to play in order to stimulate distraction and fantasy. This liberty is its
indispensable motive power and is basic to the most complex and carefully
organized forms of play."[5] The sphere of play is an excellent laboratory for
observing the peculiarities of the exocerebrum. I believe play is one of the
primordial and perhaps purest expressions of what I have called the incompleteness of the brain. Play is a useless prosthesis in its immediate expression, but it
aids in stimulating the symbolic processes of substitution. The fact that it is an
activity that humans share with the higher mammals and some birds, increases
the possibilities of analyzing the ludic phenomenon. At the biological level, play
is an activity that consumes a large quantity of energy and exposes animals to the
dangers of hurting themselves or of being surprised by a predator. However, as
the zoologist Patrick Bateson has observed, play aids in the construction of a
practical knowledge of the environment, in acquiring and perfecting physical
abilities, in consolidating social relations, and in fine-tuning both the musculature and the nervous system. Play does not have immediate functions, but in the
long term it enables young animals to simulate, in a relatively safe context,
potentially dangerous situations they may face in the future.[6]

Experiments have been conducted to prove the usefulness of play. Very
young rats were raised in total isolation; some of them had the opportunity to
play fight for one hour a day; another group was totally deprived of play. One
month later, when these rats were placed in a control rat's cage, they were
almost always attacked as intruders. The rats that had not played behaved
abnormally, with a tendency to remain motionless, unlike the rats that had had
the opportunity to play. Apparently the lack of play affected the capacity of the
rats to face a competitive world.[7] Bateson comes to the conclusion that play,
from the perspective of its function, is "developmental scaffolding"; once its
work is done, it disappears. Nevertheless, we know that play, at least in humans,
far from disappearing, remains as an important element in adult life. Therefore,
rather than a scaffold, play would be an indispensable and non-disposable
prosthesis.

---

[4] Erik H. Erikson, who was very interested in games, said that the idea of "play space" (*Spielraum*)
connotes a free movement within prescribed limits: when either the freedom or the limits end, the
game is over. See "Play and actuality," p. 133.

[5] Caillois, *Les jeux et les hommes*, p. 75.   [6] Bateson, "Theories of play," pp. 43–44.

[7] Einon and Potegal, "Enhanced defense in adult-rats deprived of playfighting experience as
juveniles." See a more recent study on play and the development of the socializing capacity in
rats: Pellis and Pellis, "Rough-and-tumble play and the development of the social brain."

I would like to go back to Piaget, who in his studies on play in children, concluded that the symbolic objects used (for example, a stick for a horse) are not only *representative* of the signified, but are also its *substitutes*.[8] For Piaget, play is essentially an assimilation of schemata of the environment; in play there is an imbalance: assimilation predominates accommodation, the latter being the modification of the schemata that are acquired for adapting to changes in the environment or to new environments. Play is a kind of ritualization of assimilated schema that goes from simple motor expression in the child to the ludic symbols of the simulated acting, when she or he feels that something can be something else.[9] In the intelligent act, according to Piaget, there is a balance between assimilation and accommodation; in contrast, in the ludic symbol the present and real object is assimilated into an anterior schema that has no objective relation to it. Imitation intervenes here as a significant gesture that evokes objects and absent schemata.[10] In this fashion, any object can be assimilated into any other one, because any thing can be the fictitious substitute of any other.[11] Thus, the object-symbol is a substitute for the signified and in this way becomes a prosthesis.

Another great psychologist, Lev Vygotsky, also asserted that play is a substitution process: it is "the imaginary, illusory realization of unrealizable desires." Vygotsky believes that play as imagination is completely absent in animals and is a specifically human form of conscious activity.[12] Even though Vygotsky supports Piaget's theses, he arrives at a different conclusion. For Vygotsky, play is never a symbolic action. He states that "the child does not symbolize in play, but desires and realizes his wishes." When a child says a stick is a horse, this is not a symbolism: "A symbol is a sign, but the stick is not the sign of a horse." And he concludes by saying that the freedom the child appears to have of voluntarily determining his or her actions is illusory, because these are subordinated to a definitive meaning, and the child acts according to the meanings of the things. Unlike Piaget, Vygotsky emphasizes the semantic dimension and does not pay attention to the symbolic elements. However, Vygotsky asserts in the same text that play is a rule that has become an affect, and he maintains that Spinoza's ideal (the concept that the affect turns into passion) "finds its prototype in play, which is the realm of spontaneity and freedom."[13]

The distinction between signs (or signals) and symbols is fundamental. Piaget, following the school of Saussure, says that a sign is a completely conventional "arbitrary" signifier determined by society. In contrast, the symbol

[8] Piaget, *La formation du symbole chez l'enfant*, p. 174.   [9] *Ibid.*, p. 98.   [10] *Ibid.*, p. 110.
[11] *Ibid.*, p. 175.   [12] Vygotstky, "Play and its role in the mental development of the child."
[13] One article that is a comparison of the thinking of Piaget and Vygotsky completely ignores the fact that the latter denied the symbolic nature of children's play. Gönzü and Gaskins, "Comparing and extending Piaget's and Vygotsky's understandings of play."

is a "motivated" signifier that has some similarity to the signified. "Symbolic play," says Piaget "poses ... the question of 'symbolic' thought in general as opposed to rational thought, whose instrument is the sign."[14] In contrast, Susanne Langer says that the symbol leads to the thinking and conceiving of the object. The sign reveals the presence of something, whereas the symbol is a tool of thought. I find Langer's definition more useful.[15]

Play is an activity that combines the symbolic peculiarities of an exocerebral prosthesis that is developed from the earliest infancy with the problems of freedom and will. Play begins as a prelingual behavior that, in my opinion, reveals how the socio-dependent neuronal networks are active from a very young age and stimulate play-oriented exocerebral chains, despite the fact that they have no immediate usefulness. Apparently there is a neuronal disposition toward play that expresses the incompleteness of the nerve circuits that are looking for external connections in order to close. In fact, children live in an essentially mimetic universe that motivates games such as those in which they pretend to be a rider, an airplane, an animal, or a car, and as the games continue they turn into more complex activities that involve the representation of characters. The psychologist Merlin Donald has developed a theory according to which the first hominids, such as *Homo erectus*, behaved like one- or two-year-old children, practically without language, but with mimetic and gesturing abilities that would have stimulated tool elaboration skills, social cohesion, and the emission of intentional vocal sounds.[16] Donald believes that it is possible that human beings that lack language are able to communicate through mimetic abilities; his examples are prelingual children, deaf individuals unable to read or write, and cases of paroxysmal aphasia. This would indicate that some primitive hominids (from the Acheulean period) had expressed themselves mimetically, but without language. There is no proof that hominids lacking language, but possessing representational mimetic capacities, existed. Nevertheless, I feel Donald's idea that establishes mimetic representation as a central factor of human society and that includes play as one of its manifestations,[17] is important.

The infantile brain attempts to complete circuits through play. By doing so, it generates symbols and converts imitation into representation. Play is stimulated by a void, due to an incompleteness, and becomes an apparently useless prosthesis, but it contributes to stimulating symbolic substitution processes. In non-human mammals there is a rudiment of this same substitution mechanism, when in their games under safe conditions, they simulate the efforts and dangers

---

[14] *La formation du symbole chez l'enfant*, p. 179.

[15] Langer, *Philosophy in a new key*. See my related comments in chapter 9 in the current volume.

[16] See Donald's books *A mind so rare*, pp. 260–261 and *Origins of the modern mind*, pp. 162ff.

[17] Donald, *Origins of the modern mind*, pp. 169–170.

of a fight or a persecution. Through the observation of play in animals, we can understand that in order for it to occur, there must be a partial deactivation of the instinctive impulses that stimulate, especially in predators, the hunting and persecution of the prey they feed on. If the instincts were not deactivated, the games would end in mortal combat, endangering the animals' lives and the survival of the species.[18] The ethologist Eibl-Eibesfeld has rightly asserted that the study of play in animals enables us to understand the distinction between non-play and play, and that it is in the latter where we demonstrate the ability to liberate ourselves emotionally from the instinctive action. Separating the ludic patterns of behavior from impulses allows us to experience play as freedom.[19] At the same time, play, in animals, is related to learning, since it helps develop abilities for capturing prey; perhaps this is why predatory mammals are the animals that play the most. But in order for play to be useful training, injuries must be kept at a minimum if instinct and emotions are unleashed during the mock combat.

According to Eibl-Eibesfeld ludic activities are separated from the neuronal mechanisms that trigger alarm, combat, and persecution under normal circumstances, and they create a stress-free emotional relaxation space. In humans, games are linked to neuronal circuits that need to be completed. It is interesting to note that laughter, which usually accompanies many games, appears to be caused by the interruption of an alarm or pain impulse. According to V. S. Ramachandran, laughter occurs when a sensation of threat or danger is blocked or aborted halfway. What causes the block is the understanding that there is no danger. If someone sits in a chair and it breaks or is rapidly removed, causing the person to end up sitting on the floor, it provokes laughter. But if in that fall, the person cracks his or her head and begins to bleed, then alarm, not laughter, is triggered. Likewise, in many games mock danger is produced, but the threat is recognized as false amid the laughter. If someone suddenly throws her or himself at us, but begins to tickle us, we burst out laughing. But if the tickling turns into punching, alarm and pain are triggered. The theory of laughter as false alarm and the origin of jokes and play are based on the study of a female patient who, when hurt, would laugh. Ramachandran proved that her pain channels were damaged. These channels begin in the insula and from there go to the anterior cingulate cortex in the frontal lobes, where the sensation of pain is felt. But this step was cut off in the patient. The insula generated the sensation of pain, but the unpleasant feeling did not follow. This interruption generated laughter.[20]

[18] The classic book on this subject is Karl Groos's, *Die Spiele der Thiere*, published in 1896. In 1899 he published another book on play in humans, *Die Spiele der Menschen*.
[19] Eibl-Eibesfeld, *Human ethology*, p. 586.   [20] Ramachandran, *The tell-tale brain*, pp. 39–40.

According to Gordon Burghardt, the peculiarities of play in animals (including humans) can be summarized into five criteria:

1. Play is a behavior that is not totally functional, directed towards stimuli that do not immediately contribute to survival.
2. Play is voluntary, spontaneous, pleasant, intentional, gratifying, fortifying, or autotelic.
3. Unlike other activities, play is an incomplete behavior, exaggerated, precocious, strange, or with known but modified patterns in its form, sequence, or objectives.
4. Play is a repeated, but not stereotyped behavior during a certain period of the animal's ontogeny.
5. Play is initiated when the animal is satisfied, fed, and protected; in other words, when it is free from fear, stress, or threats, and is not engaged in feeding, having sexual relations, or competing.[21]

Of course, in the case of non-human mammals and of birds, ludic activity is restricted to solitary rotatory or locomotive movements, the manipulation of objects, and shared social games. We do not see in them the typically human games that involve symbolic thought. However, the characteristics of play that we share with other animals are an indication that it is a very peculiar and differentiated activity that involves the somehow voluntary, but at the same time regulated, expression of functional determinants. I wish to underline the fact that play, as I mentioned before, is possibly the clearest original expression of the presence of exocerebral networks in human culture. In play, elements of what could be called a quasi-neuronal nature are combined: tension and uncertainty, repetition and rhythm, reflex and response, inhibition and discharge, excitation and delay, oscillation and synchronization. It is a revealing fact that autistic children do not have the capacity to participate in games of fantasy or imitation; the exocerebrum functions deficiently in them. An explanation of the link between games and the neuronal circuits establishes that ludic behavior is based on instinctive impulses. Roger Caillois proposed that each type of game

---

[21] Burghardt, "Defining and recognizing play." There is a very interesting precedent in the interpretation of animal play (and its relation to freedom) that is worth citing. Friedrich Schiller, in his *Letters upon the aesthetic education of man* [1794], wrote: "No doubt nature has given more than is necessary to unreasoning beings; she has caused a gleam of freedom to shine even in the darkness of animal life. When the lion is not tormented by hunger, and when no wild beast challenges him to fight, his unemployed energy creates an object for himself; full of ardour, he fills the re-echoing desert with his terrible roars, and his exuberant force rejoices in itself, showing itself without an object. The insect flits about rejoicing in life in the sunlight, and it is certainly not the cry of want that makes itself heard in the melodious song of the bird; there is undeniably freedom in these movements, though it is not emancipation from want in general, but from a determinate external necessity. The animal works, when a privation is the motor of its activity, and it plays when the plenitude of force is this motor, when an exuberant life is excited to action" (Letter 27; p. 91).

corresponds to different and powerful instincts. According to him, there would be four primary impulses in play that are the basis of games of competition, games of chance, games of simulation, and games of vertigo. Supposedly the limited, formal, and ideal satisfaction of the four instincts would be carried out in these different types of games. But if the instinct were to be extended without limits, the game would be corrupted, because that ludic behavior would invade normal daily life.[22] The result is that professional players and actors have in fact abandoned the actual sphere of play. Those who devote themselves to games of chance believing that there is a destiny that determines the results and that try in every way possible to predict them (superstitions, lucky charms, omens, methods of divination) also sidetrack the specifically ludic territory. The activities that involve vertigo, such as the mechanical rides used in fairs, the Turkish whirling dervishes, or the Mexican *voladores*, can also leave the realm of play by pursuing effects similar to those produced by drugs and alcohol. In all these cases, according to Caillois, instincts would cause the limits of the game to be overridden. But normally games discipline the instincts, even though they respond to them, and they impose an institutional existence upon them. Caillois says that from the moment games enable a formal and limited satisfaction of the instincts, "they fertilize and vaccinate the soul against their virulence."[23]

Jean Piaget rightly rejected the idea that we can find an instinct, an innate behavior, in play and in imitation, like that found in sexuality or eating. When inherited reflexes are not observed in imitation, then it is erroneously thought that they are instincts; but Piaget argues that if this were the case, then intelligence would be the most essential instinct, which he sees as a dangerous idea. This would imply regarding the very same assimilation mechanism as instinctive.[24] Piaget's fundamental conclusion is that imitation in the child is incorporated within the general schema of the sensory-motor adaptations that characterize intelligence itself.[25] On the other hand, Caillois's proposal that when play invades normal daily life it ceases to be a ludic activity contraposes the stimulating idea of Huizinga, who, with good reason, saw culture as play and warned that the ludic dimension – especially its competitive aspects – is present in political life, justice, war, poetry, philosophy, and art.

It is difficult to suppose that play is determined by instinctive impulses. Nonetheless, we can understand that ludic activity is closely linked to the neuronal circuits. What we find is a tendency to fill a void, to complete by means of imitation and play, what cannot be achieved through inborn instinctive impulses present in the cerebral networks. Caillois supposed there was some relation to the instincts; there does not appear to be any, but in contrast, there does seem to be a connection with the nervous system. A comparison could

[22] Caillois, *Les jeux et les hommes*, pp. 103–104, 113, 119.   [23] *Ibid.*, p. 121.
[24] Piaget, *La formation du symbole chez l'enfant*, pp. 81–82.   [25] *Ibid.*, p. 89.

even be made between the four impulses involved in play and certain peculiarities of the neuronal networks. Caillois speaks of four kinds of games: *agôn* (competition), *alea* (chance), *mimicry* (simulation), and *ilinx* (vertigo). These are phenomena that are not unknown to neurologists. For example, Gerald Edelman refers to the topobiological competition between neurons during the selection process that starts interlacing the neuronal networks of individuals as they grow.[26] Due to this competition, the topology of the cerebral cortex differs from one person to the next, even in the case of uniovular twins. Moreover, as Jean-Pierre Changeux has pointed out, the formation of billions of synapses in the adult brain is not entirely controlled by genes: there is a process of random variation during embryonic development that continues after birth, and that is similar to a game of trial-and-error.[27] In addition, it is possible to recognize the typical processes of simulation in certain cerebral mechanisms. The most obvious example refers to the mirror neurons that could be a neuronal correlate of the simulation process that a person needs in order to understand the minds of others.[28] And finally, I will only mention the relation between the pleasure found in vertigo or dizziness and the abuse of alcohol (and other drugs) that produces situations of tolerance and dependence.

My aim is to suggest analogies between the peculiarities of play and the neuronal networks. There are aspects of play that cannot be explained by their social or cultural function and so their connections with biological processes (instincts), or more precisely, with brain mechanisms have been looked for. However, their neuronal function is neither evident nor immediate. What is more, at first glance it could seem like a waste of time and energy, as well as a potentially risky activity resulting in injury, as the ethologist Robert Fagen has observed. "Through play," says Fagen, "the cerebral cortex is stimulated to grow, to develop, and therefore to take a larger role in control of behavior, making that behavior more flexible ... Such plasticity evolved due to the economic tradeoffs in brain development: the optimal balance between cortical and subcortical control of behavior depends on environmental information, and the experience of play reliably serves to indicate that the animal is in an appropriate environment."[29] This observation refers to animal play; in humans the symbolic dimension, which is fundamental, would naturally have to be added. But the balance that Fagen mentions makes us think that there are aspects of play that have a quasi-neuronal character and that are not completely explained simply in the context of play. These aspects, which I have already referred to, implicate an interaction between force and vacillation, reiteration and cadence, reflection and contestation, evasion and relief, provocation and

---

[26] Edelman, *Bright air, brilliant fire*, p. 83.   [27] Changeux, *L'homme de vérité*, pp. 285ff.

[28] See a good summary of this theme in Iacoboni, *Mirroring people*.

[29] Fagen, *Animal play behaviour*, pp. 19–20.

lying in wait, fluctuation and agreement. Their presence in play is better under-stood if we see them as part of a circuit that connects the cerebral networks with symbolic expressions of a cultural nature.

A ball, a pair of dice, a mask, or a swing are objects that function as powerful symbols in play, and together with the rules that direct the action, they make up a peculiar cultural prosthesis that is connected to the neuronal circuits and that is used on a soccer field, on a backgammon board, in an imaginary confrontation between cops and robbers, or at the fair. Perhaps the connection between the brain and the external symbolic circuits is more obvious in today's videogames. Here, the player literally hooks his brain up to a prosthesis (controls, a console, and a screen) manufactured by companies like Nintendo, Sega, or PlayStation. Caillois, Huizinga, or Piaget never imagined such a huge explosion of ludic alternatives as the one we are seeing in electronic and digital games. There are very complex games with highly sophisticated controls and enormous screens; there are also some that are so small that a child can take them every-where in her or his pocket. Videogames are incorporated into apparatuses (like the iPhone) that function as efficient communication means, as memories, as watches, and as interactive maps connected to global positioning systems (GPS). And one step further takes us to brain-machine connections, thanks to an implanted electrode that enables a tetraplegic person to mentally control a robotic arm. These are extremely complex prostheses that are a therapeutic expression of what I call the exocerebrum.

In 2009, Jerry Fodor, a philosopher who has supported the modular theories on brain function, criticized the ideas of Andy Clark and David Chalmers, other philosophers who had stated that electronic devices such as the iPhone form part of the mind. Fodor said that there is a gap between the mind and the world, and jokingly concluded by quoting the London Underground sign "Mind the gap," which warns passengers about the space between the train doors and the plat-form, and added that failing to do so is cause for regret.[30] According to Fodor, only that which literally does not have a derived content is mental. Given that the content of a cell phone is derived from the mind of the user, then it is not part of the mind of anybody. For him the mental is that which occurs inside the cranium. What happens outside the brain, in electronic videogames or in

---

[30] Fodor, "Where is my mind?" This is a review of Andy Clark's book, *Supersizing the mind*, which has a prologue by David Chalmers. A long time before, Gregory Bateson had laid out the problem when he asked – alluding to a blind man walking along the street with a cane – if his "self" ended at his skin or at the tip, the handle, or the middle of the cane. This question had already been posed by Maurice Merleau-Ponty in his *Phénomenologie de la perception* of 1945 (p. 179). Bateson's answer was that they all are part of an indivisible system (*Steps to an ecology of the mind*, pp. 251 and 318.) This is what is called "distributed cognition"; related to this theme, see Moreno-Armella and Hegedus, "Co-action with digital technologies," which contains a creative applica-tion to mathematics of the so-called Baldwin effect.

smartphones, is merely derived, and therefore is not mental. Apparently, for Fodor, a prosthesis would have a mental character only if it were directly implanted in the neuronal circuits. Thus, Andy Clark, in his reply to the critique, refers to a spiny lobster in a laboratory in California whose neuron in charge of rhythmic mastication was destroyed; it was replaced with a silicon circuit and the lobster recovered the atrophied function. Clark envisions a person having lost the ability to perform a simple arithmetic operation such as subtraction due to a brain injury, being connected to an external silicon circuit and recovering the lost function. Would the external circuit directly connected to that person's neurons be regarded as mental? And in another case, if the connection between the external circuit and the brain were through a portable wireless machine, would this apparatus be part of the mind?[31] What would happen if the communication were not an implant, but were auditory, visual, and tactile, as occurs with videogames and cell phones? Clark's book is a powerful, creative, and convincing defense of the idea that cognitive mental processes extend beyond the brain. For Clark, the human mind is the productive interface that connects brain, body, and the social or material world.[32]

What is important to Andy Clark to emphasize is the fact that we humans are natural cyborgs, biotechnological beings from the beginning and from birth. And so he is interested in studying the *scaffolding* that connects the body with the mind.[33] I have already mentioned that the notion of scaffolding does not seem to me to be completely adequate, given that it is a provisional structure that is installed during a construction process and removed upon its completion. What we have is more a complex technological and cultural system that is a *prosthesis* that substitutes functions that we cannot perform, or that we carry out slowly and inadequately. This system, together with the brain, is the foundation of consciousness. In contrast, Clark and Chalmers believe that the extension of the mind outside the cranium only has cognitive functions, and they are convinced that consciousness is something that occurs internally.[34] In a previous book, Clark explored the use of external symbolic structures that function better than internal computation. He stressed the resource-saving efficiency (time and work) implied in the use of external systems (such as language) but stated emphatically: "And I assuredly do not seek to claim that individual consciousness extends outside the head."[35] I believe that it does extend outside the brain, as I have extensively explained in the first part of this book.

If we see play as an exocerebral prosthesis we can understand that the extension or prolongation of mental functions into external mechanisms does not always form part of the cognitive process. Play can have some functions tied

---

[31] Letter section of the *London Review of Books*, March 26, 2009.
[32] Clark, *Supersizing the mind*, p. 219.   [33] Clark, *Natural-born cyborgs*.
[34] Clark and Chalmers, "The extended mind," pp. 223–224.   [35] Clark, *Being there*, p. 215.

to learning, but it has peculiarities that do not allow it to be understood only as a purely cognitive process. It is also the crystallization of consciousness of the self and of a free activity not determined by natural processes. There is no empty space between the videogame devices and the neuronal circuits, like the one separating the underground train from the station platform in Fodor's example. Rather, there is a continuous flow of signs and symbols between the machine and the player. In fact, in many cases the machine conducts and connects the flow between various players. The digital game devices are designed and programmed so that there is an uninterrupted communication flow between the neuronal circuits and the video-electronic systems. They are actually a very sophisticated and complex version of the former relation of players to a ball, dice, masks, or swings.

The continuous flow connecting brain and society without a doubt confronts us with very complex and thorny problems. The easy way to deal with the difficulties is simply to separate them into two spheres, as Fodor does. I would like to give another example that is more related to the theme of free will and the consequent responsibility of our acts. Michael Gazzaniga has said: "brains are automatic, but people are free."[36] Therefore, he concludes, neuroscience does not offer solutions to the problem of moral responsibility, since it only exists in the social world. Regarding play, from Gazzaniga's perspective, he would say that the brain of the player functions automatically and in a determinist manner, but in the ludic exchange there would be freedom and each participant would be responsible for the decisions made to kick a ball or to choose a mask to be a thief escaping the police. The problem with this interpretation is that it has simply separated two dimensions, the brain and society, but it does not explain the relationships between them. He says rules and values are found "*only* in the relationships that exist when our automatic brains interact with other automatic brains. They are in the ether."[37] What he finds in the ether, I believe, is the explanation of how the link between automatic organs produces free, not automatic, decisions. It is curious that he uses the old notion of ether, an invisible fluid in which the automatic cerebral apparatuses would circulate, subject to determinist rules. It is like the vehicular traffic in which physically determined devices responsibly interact; Gazzaniga says moral responsibility is a public concept that only exists in the group, not in the individual. This interpretation simply postulates that there is a void (ether) between the individual brain and society.

In contrast, Douglas Hofstadter believes that consciousness – the self – is a "strange loop" in which there is an interaction between different levels. He criticizes John Searle for wanting to locate concepts, sensations, or memory at

---

[36] Gazzaniga, *The ethical brain*, p. 99.   [37] *Ibid.*, p. 90.

the neuronal level. Hofstadter relies on Roger Sperry in order to explain that there are ideas at the higher levels of brain activity that have causal powers and they combine with other lower level forces.[38] In his famous and very imaginative book *Gödel, Escher, Bach*, he had already explained that consciousness and free will are based on a strange loop, extended as an interaction between molecular levels, signals (intermediate-level phenomena), and symbols or subsystems of the self.[39] A strange loop occurs when we move upwards or downwards through the levels of a hierarchical system, but always unexpectedly find ourselves where we first began. The key is found in the fact that in the feedback process there is a paradoxical intersection of levels.[40] The clearest examples are the drawings of Escher, some of the canons of Bach, and the incompleteness theorem of Gödel. I imagine that Hofstadter would see the interaction between the brain and the exocerebrum as a strange loop, as a feedback system that crosses different levels (molecular, neuronal, symbolic, social). It is what happens in the examples of electronic videogames: there is a flow that runs through the interface connecting the neurons of the player with the circuits of the device she or he is playing with.

McLuhan had already said this in 1969: "Now man is beginning to wear his brain outside his skull and his nerves outside his skin; new technology breeds new man." He was referring to the growing use of electronic computers, whose nature, McLuhan said, is no different from the use of ships or wheels, except in one very important aspect: previous technologies as extensions of man were fragmentary and partial, whereas the electric is total and inclusive.[41] It is an interesting observation, but he was mistaken in believing that it was in the twentieth century when humans began to use an exocerebrum. This phenomenon has existed from the very beginning, but electronics has enabled that fact to be revealed with clarity.

---

[38] Hofstatdter, *I am a strange loop*, pp. 28–32.
[39] Hofstatdter, *Gödel, Escher, Bach*, pp. 709ff.
[40] Hofstatdter, *I am a strange loop*, pp. 101–102.
[41] McLuhan, "A candid conversation with the high priest of popcult and metaphysician of media," interview in *Playboy*, March 1969.

20   External symbols

Johan Huizinga was convinced that human culture emerged from play. In his book *Homo ludens* he most emphatically stresses that he is not looking at play *in* culture, but rather is analyzing culture *as* play.[1] This is the central idea behind his study of the ludic competitions in law, war, in magic and sacred powers, in poetry, philosophy, and in art. He is especially interested in the primitive and ancient forms in which culture comes into being as play, but he also reflects on the ludic dimensions of modern culture. Huizinga can be reproached for not including a chapter on comedy, farce, and clowns. There are very few references to the theater in his work; and he does not say much about laughter, which often, though not always, accompanies play. We could say that the missing chapter had already been written by Henri Bergson, but from a very different point of view. His book on laughter, based mainly on a reflection of comedy, is also a study of the manifestations of play in the theater. For Bergson, that which is comic is an aspect of a person that makes him or her resemble something that moves rigidly, dependent on a determinism that is responsible for everything moving as if it were manipulated by wires and strings; like puppets that appear to be acting freely. However, unlike Huizinga, Bergson believes that everything that is serious in life originates in liberty, whereas play in comedy is submerged in a mechanization of life, treating life as a repetition mechanism with reducible effects and interchangeable parts.[2] For Huizinga, play, in itself, is not comic, even though he accepts that in a broad sense comic mimicry can be considered a game. In a curious book on the subject, the economist Jean Fourastié has said that laughter is a break from the determinism that constricts and limits human actions. Humor can break the determinisms and open new perspectives to the human spirit.[3]

---

[1] In the introduction to *Homo ludens* he expresses his discontent at a suggested prepositional change in the title of a conference in Zurich and in Vienna to *Des Spielelement in der Kultur*, when he did not want to use the German *in*. The same thing happened in English, with someone wanting to change his original title *The play element of culture* to *The play element in culture*.

[2] Bergson, *Le rire*, volume II, p. 1.   [3] Fourastié, *Le rire, suite.*

If we examine culture as play and play as an extension of neuronal functions, as I have proposed, we can better understand how culture, from its origin, is a strange prosthesis that completes and substitutes activities that the brain cannot perform except with the help of these external symbolic replacement networks. We can say that at the beginning of their existence, humans gambled at life and won the possibility of survival, thanks to the external ramifications of the brain. Play was a part of language and of musical and artistic manifestations. At the same time, the possibility of exercising free will was incorporated in ludic action, something that the other animals have not known, except perhaps in very limited forms.

Just as the instruments of stone, bone, or wood have been traditionally decorated with colors and symbolic drawings, so too, the construction of houses, the making of clothing, the definition of kinship systems, and the preparation of food are activities that are indissolubly linked to all kinds of symbolic encodings whose existence is not explained solely by their usefulness. They are a game and a manifestation of the exocerebral networks. They are parts of human consciousness. The decoration and incorporation of symbolic codes into instruments and daily life activities is something that is still happening today. We can ask ourselves if this intimate connection between the brain and its cultural prostheses is manifested in universal encodings that humans make from the colors, sounds, gestures, or spaces that surround them; or wonder, to the contrary, if the cultural manifestations are defined by their social context and not by the influence of inborn cerebral structures. The problem, of course, cannot be reduced to this polarity that does nothing more than force us to go back to the old polemic about which is stronger, nature or culture. As a matter of fact, we are in the presence of a continual spectrum, one in which there is no need to draw a dividing line between the brain and the exocerebrum, between the neuronal circuits and the cultural prostheses.

The idea that consciousness and the cognitive processes that accompany it form a circuit that operates not only in the brain but also in the cultural medium has often been ridiculed. Two philosophers – Fred Adams and Ken Aizawa – give an amusing example in which they compare the possibility of the existence of external circuits of consciousness and the mind with the coprophagia of certain animals.[4] In rabbits, for example, part of the digestive cycle takes place outside the body. During the first stage of digestion in the rabbit, the food, especially cellulose, is not totally decomposed. When it reaches the cecum, it is broken down by bacterial fermentation, producing the so-called cecotropes – soft, nutritious feces. The bacteria continue breaking down the elements that could not previously be digested. The animal ingests these cecotropes and in this

---

[4] Adams and Aizawa, "The bounds of cognition."

second go-around absorbs the nutrients it was unable to initially receive. Here, there is an external phase of the digestive circuit. The philosophers present this example to show that such an external phase cannot exist in cognitive processes. They believe that human beings do not excrete thoughts that can be "digested" by society in order to be reingested by internal conscious processes. Using coprophagia as a metaphor is an easy way to evoke repugnance for a process that surely has some similarity to the cecotrophy of certain rodents. The same authors give another example: it is possible to mentally calculate 347×957, by proceeding in steps, memorizing results, adding them to the next operation, and so on, until arriving at the final result. It is a laborious process; it is much easier to use a pencil and write the operations down on a piece of paper and proceed with the algorithm without the need to memorize. And using a calculator is even easier and quicker. These philosophers conclude that the paper, the pencil, or the calculator do not form part of the cognitive process; it is just the purely mental process that does so. They consider that only those processes that involve a non-derived intrinsic context can have a cognitive character. The signs written on a sheet of paper do not have a cognitive character because their significance comes from conventional associations and from the words language uses. "By contrast," they assert, "the cognitive states in normal cognitive agents do not derive their meanings from conventions or social practices."[5]

Actually, the same numbers that are "represented" in the brain and the mental algorithm used to perform the mental operation are a conventional derivation of the cultural and social context. No one without a certain education can formulate this cognitive process (347×957). No prehistoric human, for example, could work out this problem, precisely because of the inability to derive the codes of social conventions that did not yet exist. Adams and Aizawa mock the idea that a pencil thinks $347 \times 957 = 332,079$. Andy Clark answers that it is absurd to say that a pencil thinks, and not because it is derived or conventional. The pencil is simply part of a broader cognitive routine, and to suppose that it thinks is as absurd as wondering if a neuron from the parietal lobe thinks that, for example, there is a spiral in the stimulus it receives and that passes through it (and through many other neurons).[6] The resistance of Adams and Aizawa to see cultural processes as part of consciousness is symptomatic. For them, the "exograms" that Merlin Donald describes, that are external memory records, are not part of the human cognitive architecture. I can understand that my much broader idea of an exocerebrum would seem inconceivable to those who believe that no external process can form part of the circuits of consciousness.

The faith in the universality of the fundamental characteristics of human beings is frequently based on the idea that there is a general order that resides

---

[5] *Ibid.*, p. 48.   [6] Clark, *Supersizing the mind*, pp. 85ff.

only in the brain, and that confronts the existing disorder in society. The idea that there is a universal brain matter that structures the cognitive processes and behaviors is possibly a relief in light of the spectacle of a supposed growing anarchy in the world political and economic panorama. The anthropologist Emily Martin has rightly stated that instead of a social contract, which was originally seen as a way of maintaining discipline in individual rebels, today there is a chilling opposite idea: order and rationality reside in the brain and radical disorder in the social institutions.[7]

The discussion about cognitive prostheses has excessively focused on apparatuses, from cell phones with memory or calculators, to computers or photography. As I have said, I believe it is essential to add musical and artistic expressions, as well as games and speech, forms that are not such obvious instruments, like a Rolodex or a stethoscope. Even more subtle are the symbolic systems associated with kinship, food, dress, and the home; these are fundamental elements of the human daily environment and, together with language, are cultural expressions that have a universal character. Signals and marks associated with the owners of the most sophisticated and complex instruments (that house highly encoded cybernetic systems) are also usually added: cell phones or computers have individualized screens and sounds, and other instruments are painted different colors or engraved with identifying marks; even handguns or rifles frequently have ownership signs, like the bows and arrows of the past.

When we examine the classificatory logic that assigns names and functions to family members, food, clothing, or living spaces, it becomes very difficult to find universal standards. But what is definitely a generalized phenomenon is the need to encode and classify the parts of a system through symbols, whether it be one of kinship, culinary, of dress, or of housing construction. And in addition to classifying, there is a powerful impulse to not only name (an obvious necessity) but also mark, decorate, adorn, signalize, or label the components of a system. Kinship systems are not a simple cultural translation of biological events. Even though blood relationships are important, the types of relation involve a variety of codes and symbols that elude the determinants of the so-called nuclear family, made up of a woman, a man, and their progeny. In the lineal kinship systems, all the brothers and sisters of a person's parents are designated by the same two terms (uncles and aunts); and all the children of the brothers and sisters of a person's parents are called by one name (cousins). In this system, the members of the nuclear family are distinguished by sex and by generation (father, mother, daughters, sons) throughout a genealogic line traced from the mother or father (grandparents, great-grandparents,

[7] Martin, "Mind-body problems," p. 583.

grandchildren, great-grandchildren, etc.). This system, called Eskimo kinship by anthropologists, is predominant in the western world today. But it was not always so: as Jack Goody has pointed out, the European terminology went from a bifurcated collateral system to the lineal system we now use. In the former system, six functions were differentiated, with distinct names for the members of the parents' generation: father, father's brother, father's sister, mother, mother's brother, and mother's sister.[8] In Vulgar Latin the terminology changed to the lineal system at the end of the Roman era, but in Old German different names for the parent's brothers and sisters were conserved up to the sixteenth century: *Fetiro* (father's brother), *Oheim* (mother's brother), *Basa* (father's sister) and *Muoma* (mother's sister).[9]

This example that is close to us in time illustrates the importance of codes in kinship relations. The changes in European terminology that I have pointed out are related to the emergence of bilateral marriage prohibition. The terminology is associated with the inherent functions of each relative and the taboos that regulate sexual relations among them. Anthropologists have studied family and kinship structures in many different cultures in great detail. I do not want to enter into this labyrinthine theme here; I simply wish to show that, as with other aspects of human behavior, the presence of brain modules that generate certain rules in the kinship domain have been imagined. Many years ago, Dan Sperber, inspired by the ideas of Noam Chomsky, spoke of specific mental devices phylogenetically determined for the classification of kinship and of colors.[10] Modular theories have continued with this idea, and Sperber himself has decisively contributed to sustaining these interpretations.[11]

The construction and classification of living spaces are closely linked to kinship structure. Just as it is necessary to establish order in the family environment, an order that often adds artificial relations to blood relations, there is a similar need to construct and organize the environment that gives shelter and protection: the house or home. From caves or animal-skin tents to the huge

---

[8] Goody, *The development of the family and marriage in Europe*, p. 262.
[9] *Ibid.*, p. 264. See Jones, *German kinship terms (750–1500)*. In Latin, the father's sisters and brothers (*amita, patruus*) are distinguished from the mother's sisters and brothers (*matertera, avunculus*), and the descendants of the father's sisters and brothers (*patruelis*) from the descendants of the mother's sisters and brothers (*consobrinus*).
[10] Sperber, "Contre certains a priori anthropologiques."
[11] See the book by Hirschfeld and Gelman (eds.), *Mapping the mind*. Sperber has an article in this book: "The modularity of thought and the epidemiology of representations." More advanced developments in the theories on generative universal grammar have recognized a fundamental error in Chomsky's theses: his syntactocentrism. The linguist Ray Jackendoff has asserted that it nevertheless remains attached to the modular theories, and he believes at least three modules with generative capacities that are joined together by interfaces must be defined: phonological structure, syntactic structure, and conceptual structure that includes semantics (*Language, consciousness, culture*).

multifamily apartment complexes of modern cities, we find artificial environments that are built not only for protection against severe weather conditions, but also as microcosms that express and are adapted to family and tribal structures, lifestyles and religious concepts, moral habits, and esthetic tastes. Collective and private spaces are organized in houses, reflecting the prohibitions and stimuli in sexual behavior, along with the definitions of identity, shame, modesty, tolerance, and kinship. The home is a space replete with symbols, full of marks that compose a true memory archive. There is an entire universe of signs in the furniture designed for relaxation and sleep, for storing and classifying, for eating and cooking. The home is a reservoir of memories impressed into the styles and decoration of the furnishings, and the brain uses the mass of information stored in the environment. The home space is not only a memory archive; there is also a "deictic codification" process that consists of the permanent actualization of data inserted in the environment, a visual recognition through eye movements (saccadic) that absorb information imprinted in the customary environment, in the decoration of the furniture and the walls. The rapid eye movements make note of the signals in the visual field that are necessary for completing the cognition and recognition processes.[12]

The house and its furnishings, in addition to being a comfortable refuge for its inhabitants, are a cognitive prosthesis; this explains the importance – even in the simplest and poorest homes – that forms and decorations of beds, sofas, chests, wardrobes, rugs, and tapestries have had. Dining tables and chairs, so typical in the western tradition, are accompanied by very decorative crockery and cutlery.[13] It does not appear that the profusion of adornments is the manifestation of an esthetic instinct; rather, it is the expression of the cerebral circuits that are looking to be completed by all kinds of signs, symbols, and signals imprinted on the objects surrounding humans and that are usually accompanied by the appropriate ceremonial. It is interesting to see how a seventeenth-century Dutch painter, Jan Steen, paints a disorderly home as an expression of the demand for order that should prevail in houses. This order prevails in the paintings of another Dutch artist from the same period, Pieter de Hooch.[14]

When relatives sit around a table to eat, they are surrounded by objects decorated with floral, geometric, or animal motifs. The food itself, having gone through the process of cooking, also contains – along with its nutritional value – a broad set of meanings that crystallizes into the combinations of flavors. In an excellent study, Carolyn Korsmeyer has correctly stated that beyond their undeniable gustatory pleasure, tastes express meanings and therefore possess a

---

[12] Ballard, Hayhoe, Pook, and Rao, "Deictic codes for the embodiment of cognition."
[13] See Rheims, "Histoire du mobilier."
[14] See Heidi de la Mare's interesting essay, "Domesticity in dispute," in a book that explores the symbolism of the structure of homes: Cieraad (ed.), *At home.*

cognitive dimension.[15] Food forms part of a symbolic system that is very evident in religious ceremonies, but it is also observed in everyday meals.

The great classic text on taste by Jean Anthelme Brillat-Savarin, published in 1824, gives a vivid idea of the integration of food into a symbolic system: "any man who has enjoyed a sumptuous meal, in a room decorated with mirrors and paintings, sculptures and flowers, a room drenched with perfumes, enriched with lovely women, filled with the strains of soft music ... that man, we say, will not need to make too great an effort to convince himself that every science has taken part in the scheme to heighten and enhance properly for him the pleasures of taste."[16] The pleasures of food come close to other forms of integrating cultural symbols into sensations, such as takes place in the visual arts or music, associated with vision and hearing, regarded as superior senses in relation to the traditionally disdained senses of taste, smell, and touch. In the western world, the "inferior" senses are linked to potentially sinful carnal pleasures, despite their being absolutely necessary for the survival of the species. So food and sexual desire have been viewed as linked to the baser pleasures, compared with the esthetic delights provided by art and music. But, in reality, there is a convergence of the sensations that are considered spiritual, with the senses that symbolize carnality and appetites and that can degenerate into gluttony and fornication.

A peculiarity of the system of taste is the great variability in the number of taste buds in each individual; one-fifth of people are very sensitive to flavors because they have a high density of taste buds; another fifth, on the contrary, have a reduced perception of taste due to a low density of taste buds. The remainder are situated between the two extremes.[17] The diversity of what humans eat is also very great, revealing profound signs of culture and habitat in dietary customs; this diversity is based on the physiological peculiarities (omnivores) that enable the ingestion of a great variety of foods.

The sense of taste, usually linked with that of smell, channels a large number of sensations that are intermixed in the ceremonial of food and the decoration of the utensils used. Four types of taste are generally recognized: salty, sweet, sour, and bitter.[18] As in the case of the perception of colors and smells, the system of taste generates a certain encoding that separates the chemical information the taste buds receive. This is contrary to what happens in the auditory system that perceives sound wave frequencies as a flow without segmentation: the different

---

[15] Korsmeyer, *Making sense of taste*, p. 4.
[16] Brillat-Savarin, *Physiologie du goût, ou, méditations de gastronomie transcendante*, volume I, p. 68. His idea that women form part of the decoration is symptomatic.
[17] Korsmeyer, *Making sense of taste*, p. 87.
[18] Recently, the taste named *umami*, which is produced by glutamate, has been added; metallic and alkaline tastes have also been mentioned. But the definition of the basic tastes is still a matter of debate.

tones are heard in an uninterrupted sequence and their encoding appears to be entirely cultural. In the case of taste (the same as with colors and smells) there is a physiological base in the encoding that is completed by the varied cultural classification of tastes. However, the so-called basic tastes (salty, sweet, sour, and bitter) do not combine as colors do. The mixtures of primary colors produce predictable results: if red is mixed with blue, purples are produced, and if it is mixed with yellow, oranges result. But the mixture of sweet and sour substances does not produce the same results; a mixture of vinegar and honey produces a very different effect from mixing lemon and sugar in a drink. This is because the basic tastes are types that classify, whereas primary colors are wavelengths of lights and pigments. As Korsmeyer says, we cannot mix taste types, only specific substances (like honey, sugar, lemon juice, or vinegar).

Flavors, in fact, have a multisensory and interactive nature, as indicated by Gordon Shepherd.[19] Even though there is a limited number of receptors in the tongue, around a thousand nasal receptors that detect different kinds of smells must be added. Retronasal smells are those that are perceived in the back of the mouth and they combine with the primary tastes to produce many different gustatory experiences. And visual and tactile sensations are also added. Shepherd affirms that the tastes are an invention of the brain. They are certainly a combination of sensations that are culturally encoded and processed in the brain. Wine is a symptomatic and revealing example. Upon tasting it, the combination of sensations it produces is easy to confirm, not only does the retronasal smell mix with the sensations the tongue perceives, but evidently color is also an influencing factor. An experiment in 2001 with expert wine tasters was enlightening. First the different terminology to describe the flavors of the white and red wines, generally associated with fruits, was verified. Unbeknownst to the wine experts, a tasteless and odorless red dye had been added to some of the white wines. When those wines were tasted, they were described with the usual terms for red wines. Taste and smell were not determinant in the description; the visual perception associated with the culturally established codes and linked to the colors of the fruits (plums, cherries, and other similar ones) was more important.[20]

Many people have asked if the mixtures of flavors that cooking offers produce works of art similar to a poem, a sonata, or a sculpture. I find this curiosity interesting, because it gives pause for thought on the symbolic functions of food. There are those who maintain that the logic of taste differs totally from that which stimulates esthetic judgments. The basic principles of art would be completely different from the mechanisms that command taste, which are so profoundly embedded in the body that they cannot produce an esthetic emotion.

---

[19] Shepherd, *Neurogastronomy.*   [20] Morrot, Brochet, and Duboudieu, "The color of odors."

The problem would be that foods, even after very refined gastronomic treatments, do not have a meaning nor can they express emotions. Food would represent nothing beyond itself.

In my opinion food does represent something more than nutrients that are ingested; it houses meanings, expresses (and causes) emotions, and is linked to a symbolic system. This does not necessarily imply that food can be regarded as one of the arts; in my opinion, it seems that in the sense of taste there is indeed an intrinsic difficulty in generating a harmonic sequence of flavors and textures that is sufficiently fluid for producing the rapid changes comparable to those that can be perceived in music, words, and visual representation. But it is a *difficulty* not an *impossibility*. However, what interests me here is remembering what anthropologists have confirmed: that food is part of a symbolic and cognitive space. Claude Lévi-Strauss summarized it very well when he observed that natural species are not selected solely because they are "good to eat," but also because they are "good to think."[21]

The same can be said for clothing: it is crafted and chosen not only for covering, but also for thinking well. Actually, the cognitive dimension and the expression of meanings are more evident in clothing than they are in food. Besides being a protection against environmental inclemencies, clothing is a way of encoding and classifying the parts of the body, and it arises from signals that indicate what should be hidden and what can be naked, beyond the biological and climatic determinations or practical restrictions. Rules were established long ago that encoded modesty, as we call it today. The anthropologist Hans Peter Duerr has shown in his extensive investigations that the so-called process of civilization had not been gradually repressing and hiding the genital and excretory parts of the body that, supposedly in primitive, ancient, and medieval societies had been exhibited in a more natural and innocent manner. In fact, regulations that established strict codes through clothing and thereby defining nudity, modesty, and shame, have existed since ancient times.[22]

In addition to covering and hiding, clothing obviously manifests a pleasure in appearance and expresses a very diverse set of signs and symbols. Perhaps it would be excessive to say that clothing constitutes a language. But without a doubt, it contains signals that provide information as to the sex and age of a

---

[21] Lévi-Strauss, *Le totémisme aujourd'hui*, p. 132. The French philosopher Jean-Paul Jouary believes (based on Kantian categories) that cooking can come to be an art, and his example is the great Catalan chef Ferran Adrià. His cooking would result in a broadening of our knowledge of the real, in addition to being original and universal. It is difficult to give an opinion, since I have not had the opportunity to taste the art of Adrià, and I doubt I ever will (see *Ferran Adrià, l'art des mets*).

[22] Duerr, *Nudité et pudeur*. This is the first volume of a work that also explores intimacy, obscenity, and erotic love. The same theme is discussed from another perspective by Ribeiro, *Dress and morality*.

person, and frequently denotes if a female is single, virgin, married, or widowed. In different cultures, dresses show peculiar signals of a tribal, religious, hierarchal, professional, seasonal, festive, and regional nature.[23] Especially notable are the magical-religious meanings that clothes express.[24] Roland Barthes, in his stimulating reflections on fashion, disproportionately exaggerated the importance of sign in dresses. He even went so far as to assert that, "vestemes," like morphemes and phonemes in speech and language, could be defined as minimal signification units in clothing.[25] The western fascination with signals and appearances in dress can be verified in the many studies and the often lavishly illustrated books that have been dedicated to the topic. Good examples are the works of François Deserpz (1562), the Flemish engraver Abraham de Bruyn (1577), and the Italian painter Cesare Vecellio (1590); they are precursory ethnographic observations of the customs of different peoples.[26]

Thinking of dress as a language is usually connected to the idea that there is a system incorporated in some module of the brain, in which variants adapted to different cultural contexts are generated. The same thing would happen to the signs and symbols associated with kinship systems, culinary processes, and the structure of homes. Here, once again, we come up against the proposals of Noam Chomsky and the suggested alternatives of Jean Piaget.[27] From the latter's perspective, it is the construction of symbolic systems from the brain's connection with the social environment. Unlike Chomsky's innateness, in which a preformed principle responsible for the development of symbolic structures predominates, for Piaget the explanation is found rather in an epigenetic process that goes along building the symbolic systems without their having proceeded from a previously existing matrix in the brain. The use of this old contraposition (preformationism versus epigenesis), which has caused huge controversies among biologists, allows not only for the analysis of different forms of classifying the natural environment, but also the ways of interpreting the artificial structures of signs and symbols. Patrick Tort uses the dichotomy to study what he calls the "classificatory reason" that scientists have used to understand the different taxonomies and typologies that encode animal

---

[23] See Squicciarino, *Il vestito parla* and Delaporte, "Le vêtement dans les sociétés traditionelles."

[24] See Welters (ed.), *Folk dress in Europe and Anatolia*.

[25] Barthes, "La mode et les sciences humaines" and *Système de la mode*. See Yves Delaporte's comments in "Le signe vestimentaire."

[26] See Taylor, *The study of dress history*.

[27] See Royaumont's famous debate of 1975 in Piattelli-Palmarini (ed.), *Théories du langage, théories de l'apprentissage*. There Chomsky proposes to treat the problem of the nature of language in exactly the same manner that the problem of growth of a physical organ of the body is approached. For him it is the "progressive maturation of a specialized structure (hardware)." Consequently, there would be no need to speak of the "learning" of a language but of its "growth" (pp. 122–124).

species and the sciences, as well as races and social behavior.[28] He builds on a stimulating and well-known reflection of Roman Jakobson, who defined two types of verbal behavior (metaphoric and metonymic) and applied them to the comprehension of two types of aphasia (Broca's and Wernicke's). Tort believes metaphor establishes combinatory links of similarity and function according to a preformative principle that establishes internal contiguity relations. Metonymy defines epigenetic links of cause-and-effect and defines external relations. In aphasia, there would also be two poles: the disorder of the internal grammatical links and the pathology that disarticulates the relations to the external ideas and their selection. For Tort, this polarity is the same one that separates Chomsky from Piaget, innateness from constructivism, internalism from externalism, synchrony from diachrony, and preformation from epigenesis.[29]

From Piaget's perspective, and continuing Huizinga's interpretation, we can understand that there are important ludic elements in the crystallization process of symbols in dress, the home, food, and kinship. Necessity is not the only thing that propels the incorporation of symbols and signs into a dinner, a dress, or the definition of kinship rules. There is also free and pleasurable play that interweaves norms and diversion, as also happens in music, dance, painting, or literature.

The symbolic systems are only partially housed in the brain. They are principally structures that have gone along being built not just as a social expression of cerebral modules, but as the product of an intense interaction between the socially dependent neuronal systems and the cultural textures surrounding people. It is a self-regulation process. The external symbolic textures are continuously created and used – consciously or unconsciously – by the neuronal circuits that cannot function adequately without these prostheses.[30] When individuals are inclined to make a decision, they take time, sometimes a

---

[28] Tort, *La raison classificatoire*. See Roman Jakobson, "Two aspects of language and two types of aphasic disturbances."

[29] Piaget believed there were parallels between phylogeny and ontogeny, having been influenced in his youth by the ideas of Haeckel, while studying paleontology (his thesis was a study on Jurassic gastropods). The great biologist Stephen Jay Gould wrote him in 1972 asking his opinion of Haeckel's work. Piaget answered that he had done little psychological research on the relationship between ontogenesis and phylogenesis, but that he believed that the child explained more to the adult than vice versa. Gould contends that Piaget remained situated between two extremes: between the neo-preformativism of Chomsky and the old theories of the blank slate. Gould emphatically affirms that phylogeny does not cause ontogeny, although there are parallels. See Gould, *Ontogeny and phylogeny*, pp. 144–147.

[30] J. Kevin O'Regan has explained, from the neuroscientific and psychological perspective, this function of the external prostheses very well: "seeing constitutes an active process of probing the external environment as though it were a continuously available *external memory*. This allows one to understand why, despite the poor quality of the visual apparatus, we have the subjective impression of great richness and 'presence' of the visual world: But this richness and presence are actually an illusion, created by the fact that if we so much as faintly ask ourselves some question

very long time, to think about and weigh the alternatives. Of course, this "thinking" involves deliberation with other people in the framework of institutions that are subject to rules. But it is also an individual meditation that naturally includes the application of a certain degree of rationality. And added to that is a thoughtful examination that mixes the ideas flowing from the brain with the absorption of sensations and signals that proceed from the symbolic systems surrounding us, incorporated into the rooms of the house, the flavors of the food, the music we listen to, the texts we read, the sites we visit on the Internet, the familiar objects that surround us, or the clothes we wear. We are wrapped in a set of textures, smells, sensations, emotions, flavors, sounds, images, and words that transmit signs and symbols. Even though they proceed from structured systems, the flow of signals we are immersed in can be chaotic or tumultuous; the person that digresses while meditating upon the decision that needs to be made is submerged in that flow. Here, there is literally a game with the waves of the external symbols that bathe individuals the entire time they are awake. People consciously or unconsciously use parts of that symbolic bath to stimulate reflection.

We can ask ourselves: does this deliberate meditation, though digressive and ludic, interrupted by moments of more systematic and even rational reflection, allow us to make voluntary and free decisions? Can the deliberation and discussion with other people, combined with contemplative reveries in which our thoughts meander through the environment, be part of the exercise of free will? My answer is yes. This game that joins the activity of the brain with the symbolic circuits of the environment opens the possibility of making voluntary decisions that elude determinist chains. Play breaks the chain of determinations. In this way we can understand that free will has its roots in culture and, as a consequence, there are diverse forms of freedom.

about the environment, an answer is immediately provided by the sensory information on the retina, possibly rendered available by an eye movement." ("Solving the 'real' mysteries of visual perception," p. 484).

21   Final reflections

The excursion through the small world that surrounds us, the world of the family, the home, food, and dress helps us understand the immediacy of the swarm of symbols that envelops us. This immediacy is not so evident in the great social theater, where powerful institutions and strong confrontations – though replete with symbols – disconcert us with their thunderous spectacle. It is a paradoxical spectacle of technological progress and misery, of wealth and of wars, of massive communication and loneliness, of political celebrities and famous stars, of judgments and crimes.

The small world that environs us is very similar to the world surrounding the animals – the *Umwelt* – that the Estonian biologist Jakob von Uexküll, today regarded as the founder of biosemiotics and to whom I briefly referred in chapter 3, defined and studied. For Uexküll each animal species has its own *Umwelt* that, in turn, is made up of two worlds respectively connected to a receptor system and an effector system. The first (the *Merkwelt*) is a set of signs that the organism is capable of perceiving, and the second (the *Wirkwelt*) is the part of the world that is capable of affecting. So there is a world composed of objects to which the animal can pay attention and another world composed of the objects that can be affected by the action of the organism. Together they form an animal's *Umwelt*. Uexküll describes the overlapping of different *Umwelten* as follows:

Let us examine, for instance, the stem of a blooming meadow flower and ask ourselves which roles are assigned to it in the following four environments: (1) in the environment of a flower-picking girl who is making a bouquet of colorful flowers and sticking it as a decoration on her bodice; (2) in the environment of an ant, which uses the regular pattern of the surface of the stem as the ideal paving to get to its feeding area in the flower's leaves; (3) in the environment of a cicada larva, which bores into the vascular system of the stem and uses it as a tap in order to build the liquid walls of its airy house; (4) in the environment of a cow, which grabs both stem and flower in order to shove them into her wide mouth and consume them as feed.[1]

---

[1] Uexküll, *Meditaciones biológicas*, p. 24.

Thus, concludes Uexküll, the same flower stem plays a different role in each *Umwelt*; an adornment, a pathway, a deposit, or food. The objects (like the stem) are signs and because of them, according to his famous phrase, "no animal ever appears as an observer; one may assert that no animal ever enters into a relationship with an 'object'. Only through the relationship is the object transformed into the carrier of a meaning that is impressed upon it by a subject."[2] This formulation would have delighted the structuralist semiologists like Roland Barthes.

The importance of the concept of the *Umwelt* is the fact that it conceives of the organism in its unit with an environment made up of objects that are carriers of meaning. When Uexküll refers to the perception world (the *Merkwelt*) of humans, he concludes that "it is a living part of us."[3] He also asserts that the perception world is the equivalent of the psychologists' concept of psyche.[4] He maintains that it is advantageous to substitute the psyche with the *Merkwelt*, because the psyche impedes the introduction of the question of free will and what is beautiful in the animal world. I believe that this idea of the surrounding world (which is part of what I call the exocerebrum) makes it possible to present the problem of human free will in such a way that it can have a solution. Naturally, this is a meaningless matter in relation to animals.

It is interesting to note that Uexküll was the source of inspiration for the Spanish philosopher José Ortega y Gasset in formulating his famous maxim "I am I and my circumstance, and if I do not save it, I do not save myself," in his book *Meditaciones del Quijote*, written in 1914. In it, Ortega refers to his environment, the mountains of Guadarrama and the fields of Ontígola, and says that this "surrounding reality forms the other half of my person" and through it "I can integrate myself and be completely myself." Although he does not say so here, it is obvious that his thought is based on the ideas of the *Umwelt* developed by Uexküll: "The most recent biological science," Ortega says, "studies the living organism as a unit composed of the body and its particular environment, in such a way that the vital process does not consist only of an adaptation of the body to its environment, but also of the environment to its body."[5] In 1922 Ortega himself published Uexküll's *Bausteine zu einer biologischen Weltanschauung* with a presentation of his in which he says "these biological meditations have had an influence on me since 1913."[6] The concept of the *Umwelt* is closely tied to the idea that consciousness is not only an "I"

[2] *Ibid.*, p. 19.   [3] Uexküll, *Ideas para una concepción biológica del mundo*, p. 231.
[4] *Ibid.*, p. 72.   [5] Ortega, *Meditaciones del Quijote*, pp. 76–77.
[6] Published in the *Biblioteca de Ideas del Siglo XX* directed by Ortega. The footnotes written by Julián Marías, in the 1957 edition of *Meditaciones del Quijote* give a detailed explanation of Uexküll's influence on Ortega. The Spanish anthropologist Julio Caro Baroja was also familiar with the work of Uexküll and commented on it in his book *Los Baroja*, p. 87. See Utekhin, "Spanish echoes of Jakob von Uexküll's thought."

floating around in the brain, but that it also includes the environment. It was an idea that captivated Ortega, who might have exclaimed: I am I and my *Umwelt*.

The idea that the self is not just embedded in the body but that it also forms part of a surrounding world came to be accepted by various thinkers. At the end of the seventeenth century, John Locke stated that the person – the self – is a concept that implies a forum: in other words, a social environment.[7] Later, Jean-Jacques Rousseau critically saw human existence as dependent on the social environment: "the savage lives within himself: the social man is always outside of himself and does not know how to live outside the opinion of others, and from this unique judgment, to put it like that, he obtains the sensation of his own existence."[8]

Closer to us in the nineteenth century, the novelist Henry James, through a character (Madame Merle) in *The portrait of a lady* (1881), vividly expressed the idea that the self extends into the surrounding world:

When you've lived as long as I, you'll see that every human being has his shell and that you must take the shell into account. By the shell I mean the whole envelope of circumstances. There's no such thing as an isolated man or woman; we're each of us made up of some cluster of appurtenances. What shall we call our "self"? Where does it begin? Where does it end? It overflows into everything that belongs to us – and then it flows back again. I know a large part of myself is in the clothes I choose to wear. I've a great respect for *things*! One's self – for other people – is one's expression of one's self; and one's house, one's furniture, one's garments, the books one reads, the company one keeps – these things are all expressive.[9]

Of course Uexküll would not have much liked this emphasis on the relation of the human animal to *things*. In his theory of the *Umwelt*, the important aspect is that these things function as signs or symbols, not as objects. But he would have recognized the *significant* dimension of the things that Henry James emphasized. It is interesting that Henry's brother, William James, expressed exactly the same idea in *The principles of psychology* from 1890: "*In its widest possible sense*, however, *a man's Self is the sum total of all that he* CAN *call his*, not only his body and his psychic powers, but his clothes and his house, his wife and children, his ancestors and friends, his reputation and works, his lands and horses, and yacht and bank account. All these things give him the same emotions."[10]

I have quoted these lines here because they bring us closer to the idea of an "I" that extends out into the nearby, and even intimate, environment, which functions as an exocerebrum and enables us to understand the concrete conditions on

[7] Locke, *An essay concerning human understanding*, chapter 27, §§ 23–27.
[8] Rousseau, *Discours sur l'origine et les fondemens de l'inegalité parmi les hommes*, p. 193.
[9] Henry James, *The portrait of a lady*, pp. 259–260.
[10] William James, *The principles of psychology*, p. 291.

which self-consciousness is based. The most abstract expressions of this *Umwelt* can make us lose sight of the everyday referents. This notion was not only adopted by biology; for example, it was also a fundamental part of the phenomenology of Edmund Husserl, an idea that did not proceed from Uexküll and that I will not go into here. But I will briefly refer to some direct philosophical repercussions of Uexküll's theses. They were used by Martin Heidegger, for example, in a course he gave on metaphysics in Freiburg in the winter 1929–30 semester. Heidegger praises Uexküll for his investigations on the relation of the animal to its surrounding environment and comments that they also interest him for being a sharp criticism of Darwinism. For Heidegger the *Umwelt* is what he calls the "disinhibiting ring"; disinhibition is what enables an organism to be capable of a conduct that is motivated inside its world or ring. But Heidegger believes that the surrounding human world is very different from that of the animal, and that it is not simply a qualitative otherness (even less so a quantitative one) of what is human in the face of what is animal. Rather it is a question of knowing "if the animal has the capacity to apprehend something *as* something." The animal is not capable of that and therefore "is separated from man by an abyss."[11] In animals there is what is called a "poverty in world" because they are not capable of knowing things as things, whereas humans are formers or shapers of world. This is one of the bases for thinking of the human as an opening, as a being-in-the-world.

Several years later, in 1944, Ernst Cassirer retook the ideas of Uexküll to support his idea of humans as "symbolic animals." Both had been professors at the University of Hamburg at the same time in the 1920s. In 1933 Uexküll gave a conference there on the olfactory field in dogs. Cassirer, who was attending, intervened to point out that Rousseau had stated that the first man to have built a fence, declaring "this is mine," should have been killed. He then added that this would not have been enough: it ought to have been extended to the first dog, too. And regarding dogs, it should be mentioned that Joseph Goebbels, Hitler's propaganda minister, was also in the audience. That same year Cassirer fled Hamburg due to the anti-Jewish atmosphere that was palpable in the universities (Uexküll apparently defended him). Cassirer understood that the idea of Umwelt is not a psychological interpretation, but a concept based on the strict observation of the anatomic structure and behavior of animal species. There is a coordinated balance between the receptor and effector worlds; Cassirer believed that there is a qualitative change in the functional circle (the Umwelt) of human beings that makes it different from the world surrounding animals: the symbolic system incorporated by language, myth, and religion has to be considered. The human experience is enveloped in a complex symbolic network. Therefore,

---

[11] Heidegger, *The fundamental concepts of metaphysics*, § 61, b. An interesting reflection on Uexküll and Heidegger can be seen in Agamben, *The open*.

Cassirer prefers to define humans as symbolic animals rather than rational animals. In the world that surrounds animals, there are only signals; in the world surrounding humans, there are symbols. And so for Cassirer, the closed functional circle of the animal *Umwelt* is a concept that is not applicable to humans. Nevertheless, Cassirer did not examine the possibility of a symbolic *Umwelt* as an extension of the brain through which the relation between the mind and the cultural environment could be explored.[12]

Another philosopher, Maurice Merleau-Ponty, in his course from 1957–58, took Uexküll's theories as a point of support to explain the "architecture of symbols" that even in non-human animals appears as a kind of "pre-culture"; this occurs when the *Umwelt* becomes increasingly less directed toward a finality and more toward the interpretation of symbols. In the *Umwelt* there is not just the sum of exterior events or a relation to the interior subjective space. Merleau-Ponty affirms that human consciousness is a "transcendental field"; the human *Umwelt* is an open field that is not a product of freedom in the Kantian sense (that is to say, as a free event linked to a decision); it is more a structural freedom, in the sense of how Uexküll understands the *Umwelt*: like a melody in which we no longer can see the organism – in its relation to the exterior world – as an effect of that external environment, nor as its cause.[13]

Certainly, the problem of liberty is inserted into that open field that is the world surrounding humans. The notion of *Umwelt* enables the problem and the parameters that define it to be situated, but Uexküll's interpretation is too anchored in the old vitalism, in an outdated antievolutionism and a metaphysical vision to constitute enough of a base for resolving the problem. From another perspective, the great economist and liberal philosopher Friedrich August Hayek, opponent of the Keynesian theses, took the matter on. Hayek was first educated as a psychologist and in the 1920s he wrote an essay that he never published, in which he proposed a theory that advances ideas that were discussed much later on. He also introduced a hypothesis that was developed afterward by Donald Hebb (in 1964) on how neuronal activity strengthens certain synaptic connections for recording memory, which was an exhibition of brain plasticity.[14] In 1952, Hayek published his book *The sensory order*, taken from his youthful manuscripts. It is very interesting to see how the great defender of modern freedom tackled the problem of free will from a psychological and philosophical perspective. To begin with, Hayek asserts that there is no isomorphism between the physical order of the external world and the

---

[12] Cassirer, *An essay on man*, chapter 2; Heusden, "Jakob von Uexküll and Ernst Cassirer." Also see Weber, "Mimesis and metaphor." Jürgen Habermas refers to Uexküll in his interesting text on Cassirer and Gehlen: "Symbolic expression and ritual behavior."

[13] Merleau-Ponty, *Nature*, pp. 167–178 and 198.

[14] A good general view of the topic of plasticity can be read in Doidge, *The brain that changes itself.*

sensory order (mental or phenomenic). In contrast, he proposes that there is identity, rather than isomorphism, between the sensory or mental order and the neuronal order.[15] I suppose he uses the concept of isomorphism more as a metaphor than as a rigorous mathematic (or mineralogic) notion for referring to the similarity between the forms or structures of phenomena or things of different origin. In any case, Hayek posits a world-mind duality that does not help understand the problem of free will and that is opposed to the idea of an *Umwelt* structurally linked to the individual. Hayek realizes that biology does not allow him to understand the responses to external stimuli that are directed toward ends, responses that are characteristic of the most developed central nervous systems. However, he vaguely turns to concepts of homeostasis and open systems developed by Walter B. Cannon and Ludwig von Bertalamffy. But he comes up against a serious problem when, despite denying the differences between neuronal and mental order, he feels obligated to adopt a dualist vision.[16] Since the unification of mental events and physical events seems impossible to him, he has no choice but to accept what he calls a "practical dualism" based on the assertion of an objective difference between the two types of events, and especially on the demonstrable limitations of the powers of our mind to understand the unitary order they belong to.

For Hayek every concept of a mind explaining itself is a logical contradiction and he is convinced that it will never be possible to build a bridge across the space between the spheres of the mental and the physical.[17] Arriving at this point, Hayek runs into another problem, that of free will: "Even though we may know the general principle by which all human action is causally determined by physical processes, this would not mean that to us a particular human action can ever be recognizable as the necessary result of a particular set of physical circumstances. To us human decisions must always appear as the result of the whole of a human personality – that means the whole of a person's mind – which, as we have seen, we cannot reduce to something else."[18] This means that free will only depends on the acceptance of a "practical dualism," but such a duality – in a unified vision – does not actually exist. In a note to this statement Hayek says that the word "free" has been formed to describe a given subjective experience and that it can barely be defined, except in reference to that experience, and at most, it could be said to be a meaningless term. But this would imply, he believes, that any denial of free will would be as absurd as saying it existed.

A few years later in his celebrated book *The constitution of liberty* (1960), Hayek repeated his idea about free will: it is a phantasmal problem whose affirmation or denial is senseless. However, after discussing voluntarist and

---

[15] Hayek, *The sensory order*, §§ 2.7, 2.8, and 2.10.   [16] *Ibid.*, § 8.46.
[17] *Ibid.*, §§ 8.90 and 8.91.   [18] *Ibid.*, § 8.93.

determinist ideas he is clearly inclined toward the former: "the voluntarists are more nearly right, while the determinists are merely confused."[19]

Since for Hayek, the problem amounted to understanding how the exterior world is represented, reproduced, and classified in the human mind, he inevitably arrives at an infinite regression, belonging to the old idea of the homunculus: the reproduction of the reproduction that, in turn, must include a reproduction of that reproduction, and so on, *ad infinitum*. This is the reason why Hayek believes it is impossible to totally comprehend the surrounding external world.[20] Coming to this conclusion, the great liberal evaded the possibility of securing the notion of liberty to a solid scientific base.

The problem of the "unification" of the mental and neuronal orders cannot be thought of as *reducing* the conscious to the physical order, because all reduction leads to the absurd. The same thing happens when *increasing* or *elevating*, so to speak, the physical order to the social sphere: it is absurd to explain the results of the investigation in physics, as mere social or cultural constructions. This cognitive relativism is as damaging as the reductionism that crushes the dynamics of consciousness on a rigid monistic determinism.

The reflections of Hayek were picked up by another great economist, Douglass North (he too, a Nobel laureate), who by understanding economy as a theory of choice, has gotten closer to the neuronal questions. From this concept of economy, North is interested in the "intentionality of the players" and in the surrounding cultural world in whose context the decisions are made. In his pioneering study on the sensory order, Hayek rightly states that our knowledge is, at best, fragmentary; but he was mistaken in not understanding that it is necessary to carry out processes of "social engineering," even though he was correct in his discussion with the socialist planners. This leads North to underline the importance of conscious human intentionality and to maintain that it is embodied in the social institutions. The difficulty lies in the fact that decisions and choices occur in what he calls a non-ergodic world – that is, a social world in continuous change and full of uncertainty. The decisions are inserted in a cultural space in which many different belief systems coexist that combine both rational and irrational attitudes. North recognizes that Hayek understood that the mind is inseparably connected to the environment and that it builds classificatory systems to understand it. From this point, North relies on Merlin Donald, whom I mentioned in chapter 5, to recognize the tremendous influence of the symbolic environment.[21]

In my opinion, the uncertain cultural environment forces human beings to constantly make decisions. But at the same time, the symbolic world that

---

[19] Hayek, *The constitution of liberty*, pp. 135–136, in chapter 5.
[20] Hayek, *The sensory order*, § 8.9.
[21] North, *Understanding the process of economic change*, p. 34.

surrounds them opens up the possibility of escaping from the determinist biological space to enter into a world in which it is possible, though difficult, to
choose freely. Of course, the sociocultural world is not a contingent space in
which options randomly arise in the presence of stunned humans who would
have to make decisions in a space that not only was uncertain, but also
incomprehensible. From a biological point of view, the relation of humans to
the surrounding world is frequently interpreted as a homeostatic phenomenon.
Homeostasis (*homeo* = similar, *stasis* = stability) functions the same in a
unicellular being, like the amoeba, as it does in organisms as complex as the
higher mammals. It is a tendency that keeps the interior environment of animals
stable, through physiological processes that interact with the exterior.

The neurologist Antonio Damasio, for example, believes that homeostasis is
the model that explains the attitudes and actions characteristic of conscious
minds, which create new forms of reaching a stable balance at the level of
the sociocultural spaces.[22] Just as the imbalances in the internal environment
are corrected thanks to homeostatic impulses, the social imbalances would
be compensated through, for example, moral rules and laws. According to
Damasio, there would be a sociocultural homeostasis that would function
essentially like that of the amoebas.[23] Human consciousness would function
as a thermostat, so to speak, capable of regulating the temperature of an
environment, but at a much more complex level. Political and economic
systems, the same as scientific activity, would respond to functional problems
of the social space that need to be corrected and balanced. For Damasio,
sociocultural homeostasis would be the continuation, at a high level of complexity, of the same mechanism that regulates the life of unicellular organisms.
In these organisms the process is automatic, whereas in beings that are conscious of automatism, the influence of self-oriented deliberation is added.[24] The
Umwelt model formulated by Uexküll has the advantage of explaining the
relation of the organism to its symbolic environment as a semiotic space. But
it has the great disadvantage, due to Uexküll's stubborn antievolutionism, of
rejecting the idea of adaptation in the name of a supposed perfect balance
between the animal and its environment. In contrast, homeostasis implicates a
continuous adaptation of the organism to provoked imbalances, such as the
scarcity of food, the lack of water, or the rigors of climate.

But it is my opinion that in order to understand the phenomenon of human
consciousness, a very important piece must be added to Damasio's proposal. It
is necessary to consider the great leap that resulted in the emergence of a hybrid
and heterogeneous interior environment in humans. Unlike the other animals,
humans have to maintain an internal medium that is also external, in the sense

---

[22] Damasio, *Self comes to mind*, p. 26.   [23] *Ibid.*, p. 292.   [24] *Ibid.*, p. 176.

that the brain receives the intrusion of exogenous artificial elements. This hybrid and heterogeneous condition is what enabled the development of self-consciousness. So it seems pertinent to me to borrow another medical term, *heterostasis*, to refer to the tendency to maintain a relative balance in the presence of the heterogeneity of elements in the circuits of consciousness. I am referring to the existence of a symbolic substitution system connected to the neuronal networks; in other words, to the coexistence of cultural prostheses and cerebral networks in one and the same space.

The concept of heterostasis was proposed in 1973 by the Hungarian endocrinologist Hans Selye, as a complementary process to homeostasis. In this process the organism suffers a systemic adaptation in the presence of toxic exogenous substances.[25] This stimulates hormonal mechanisms that allow the foreign element to be tolerated without attacking it, or destroying only its excess.[26] Thus, a new balance is established between the body and the exogenous substances. To describe this process Selye spoke of heterostasis (*heteros* = other, *stasis* = stability). Homeostasis maintains a stable atmosphere in relation to a "normal" point, whereas heterostasis changes that point due to the exogenous intervention. This is what usually happens when the organism adapts to high levels of alcohol, drugs, or poisonous contaminants, by increasing tolerance in response to toxins. The new balance implies that the body now depends on the presence of the foreign elements.

Something similar must have occurred when primitive humanity adapted to the changes in the surrounding world, thanks to the use of the new symbolic prostheses such as speech, painting, music, and the semantic elements associated with cooking, housing, and dress. All this, of course, was added to the fabrication and use of instruments made of stone, wood, and bone that were a valuable prolongation of the hands. Paradoxically, these prostheses were developed thanks to a dependence of the brain that not only became addicted to them, but that adapted to the new situations by virtue of the fact that a new balance was established with the artificial part of its surrounding world. It was a process of heterostasis that resulted in what I call the socio-dependency of certain neuronal circuits, brought on by their incompleteness. The strange paradox is that thanks to this dependency of external symbolic circuits, the door to free will was opened, as if the exocerebral prostheses were a kind of liberating drug and not an enslaving chain. A brain that is subject to the cultural networks opens the doors to freedom.

---

[25] Selye, "Homeostasis and heterostasis." See also Berntson and Cacioppo, "From homeostasis to allodynamic regulation."

[26] This is referring to syntoxic (an increase in tissue resistance) and catatoxic (elimination of the excess toxic elements) actions. Heterostasis is also called allostasis.

Another example of modification of the internal physiological medium caused by an external prosthesis is what Stanislas Dehaene defined as a process of neuronal reconversion. When a person reads, a small region in the left ventral visual pathway of the brain is always activated. It is the area in charge of the visual form of words, and it is located in exactly the same place, with millimetric variations, in all people of all cultures. Dehaene explains that since writing is a recent invention, it cannot be thought that the brain adapted to it during the course of evolution. What happened is that the learning of writing recycled a region of the brain whose initial function was similar; it is a process that resembles the exaptation described by Stephen Jay Gould.[27] According to Dehaene's hypothesis, cultural objects must find an "ecological niche" in the brain: a circuit or a set of circuits whose original function is used and whose flexibility is sufficient for its being reconverted into a new function.[28] Here, writing and reading are the liberating drugs the brain becomes addicted to, that modified its homeostatic balance in order to enable the functioning of a hybrid structure based on a feedback system: a loop that includes neuronal circuits and cultural networks and that ensures a constant back-and-forth between the symbolic cultural environment and the central nervous system. This hybrid structure becomes autonomous and can be responsible for the acts it causes. The example of reading and writing is revealing because it involves a process of liberation: the hybrid mechanism allows there to be creative acts that are not inserted in an inexorable chain of cause and effect. Literature, like other artistic expressions, is a liberating activity. The hands of the writer are not like those of Orlac, subject to a determinant power alien to consciousness. The hands of the writer are a means of liberation.

In finishing, I invite the reader to take a look back at the different topics covered in this final part. It is worth remembering some of the nodal points and how they connect with one another in a line of argument. I have explained how consciousness, understood as an impulse through which people become aware of their "I," forms part of a circuit that is not housed solely inside the brain. It is a hybrid circuit similar to what Spinoza called *conatus*, and it is here that the so-called will is capable of modifying the same neuronal networks that seem to determine its behavior. Free will, a scarce good, is possible precisely thanks to the exocerebral networks that are responsible for the singularity that is present only in humans and that ensures the coexistence of indeterminism and deliberation. The door is now opened to behaviors that are neither random, nor determined by a cause-and-effect chain firmly fixed in the brain. Consequently,

---

[27] The process of exaptation is the refunctionalization of the non-adaptive modifications Gould calls *spandrels* that I mention in chapter 2.

[28] Dehaene, "Les bases cérébrales d'une acquisition culturelle," p. 198.

we cannot accept the idea that there is a moral module in the central nervous system capable of determining the ethical decisions of individuals. This proposal, which is a mechanical transfer of Chomsky's ideas on generative grammar to the field of morality, lacks a scientific base and denies the possibility of free will. Liberty is based on the presence of artificial cultural prostheses (firstly language) that substitute functions the brain cannot carry out through exclusively biological means. The nervous circuits need an exocerebrum in order to operate to their fullest capacity. The exploration of certain facets of this exocerebrum shows that the possibility of free will resides in its operation. One of the most significant and revealing aspects analyzed is that of play, an activity that is characterized by the combination of rules and freedom. The ideas of Huizinga, Caillois, and Piaget show how play is a behavior that escapes from determinism and is stimulated by that incompleteness typical of the human brain, which makes it dependent on cultural and social structures. This dependency, paradoxically, opens a slit through which free will enters. Another exploration makes it possible to illustrate the peculiarities of a surrounding world, very near and routine, in which the symbolic structures crystallize into kinship systems, the home, dress, and cooking. These structures envelop us in networks that instead of trapping us, set us free; they define our individuality and our inclusion in a cultural conglomerate.

But this is where a doubt arises. We can understand that speech, the arts, and music have a liberating role, even though their rules and structures also restrict our acts. If they did not restrict them, the freedom would be meaningless. Nevertheless, the prostheses that surround us and envelop us have grown to such an exorbitant extent that we have to wonder if this expansion will change the conditions that allow there to be free will. Electromechanical and digital supports are growing in a way that to many seems monstrous. The exocerebrum is becoming robotized and automatized. We live surrounded by apparatuses that are increasingly smarter and more sophisticated. The technologies that produce rapid and wide-spectrum interfaces connecting the human brain with machines advance on a daily basis. Buildings and transportation means are beginning to be made with materials and devices that have abilities to adapt to changing situations without our intervention. Robots and computerized mediums have appeared that are capable of acquiring a certain degree of personality and have developed states of alert and attention similar to humans. Thanks to nanotechnology, new forms of dress, with computational capacities and automatic adaptation processes, could soon become intelligent body wrappings. Even cooking could be converted into a product of chemical combinations controlled by computers and automated machines. In the not-too-distant future, the robotic construction of extraterrestrial bases will proceed and perhaps begin to exploit the resources on the Moon, on some satellites, and on Mars. That surely will require robots capable of programming themselves and other robots.

If at times the things that surround us – the instruments, clothing, furniture – seem oppressive merely by their presence, if fashions and novelties harass and appear to dominate us, what can we expect from a prosthetic environment as highly sophisticated and intelligent as the one developing today? There are those who fear, perhaps influenced by science fiction, that the prostheses will eventually control us. Is it possible that a dramatic inversion could occur in such a way that our brains end up being the somatic prostheses of some complex cybernetic structures? For that to happen, there would have to be a spectacular revolution: that the apparatuses possessing artificial intelligence were able to develop a consciousness and a freedom sustained by the neuronal networks of their former masters (as happened with the computer HAL in Kubrick's movie *2001: A space odyssey*, from 1968). Humans are provided with consciousness thanks to the prostheses they create. There is a fear that the prostheses – which are increasingly faster, more intelligent, and more rational – take the leap and acquire the capacity to be self-conscious. And that they do so at the cost of converting humans into biological prostheses, in a process similar to the one we followed to develop a non-organic exocerebrum.

Our imagination can carry us far away, but today we only have stories of robots with a very limited capacity and that are very far from attaining humanoid forms of consciousness and free will. The cyborgs of today, for their part, are simply humans with implants that do not appear to have any power over the body. Undoubtedly, it is the surprising results of very advanced technologies we are concerned with, and everything points to their unrestrained development in the coming decades. In order to understand the challenges that await us in light of these technological advances, it is advisable for us to reflect carefully on our ancient relation to the prostheses and artifices that made us self-conscious humans with the capacity to choose freely. This is what I have proposed to do in these pages. If we are to imagine cybernetic machines that manage to attain their liberty and their autonomy, breaking the chains that hold them to humans, we must first think about the conditions that allow us to be free. Machines, today, still constitute a world that is completely dominated by determinist chains, except when their inventors exercise the free will that, with much difficulty, they have acquired.

Bibliography

Adams, Fred and Ken Aizawa. "The bounds of cognition," *Philosophical psychology* 14 (1) (2001): 43–64.

Addis, Laird. *Of mind and music*, Ithaca: Cornell University Press, 1999.

Agamben, Giorgio. *The Open: Man and Animal*, Stanford: Stanford University Press, 2004.

Álvarez Buylla, Arturo and Carlos Lois. "Mecanismos de desarrollo y plasticidad del sistema nervioso central," in Ramón de la Fuente and Francisco Javier Álvarez Leefmans (eds.), *Biología de la mente*, Mexico: Fondo de Cultura Económica, 1998, pp. 105–146.

Álvarez Leefmans, Francisco Javier. "La conciencia desde una perspectiva biológica," in R. de la Fuente (ed.), *Aportaciones recientes de la biología a la psiquiatría*, Mexico: El Colegio Nacional, 2003.

Álvarez Leefmans, Francisco Javier. "La emergencia de la conciencia," in R. de la Fuente and F. J. Álvarez Leefmans (eds.), *Biología de la mente*, Mexico: Fondo de Cultura Económica, 1998.

Andrews, Kristin. "Review of Neurophilosophy of free will," *Philo* 6 (1) (2003): 166–175.

Anzieu, Didier. *Le moi-peau*, Paris: Dunod, 1995.

Aunger, Robert. "Culture vultures," *The Sciences* 39 (5) (1999): 36–42.

Aunger, Robert. *The electric meme: A new theory of how we think*, New York: The Free Press, 2002.

Axel, Richard and Linda Buck. "A novel multigene family may encode odorant receptors: A molecular basis for odor recognition," *Cell* 65 (1991): 175–187.

Bach-y-Rita, Paul. *Brain mechanisms in sensory substitution*, New York: Academic Press, 1972.

Bach-y-Rita, Paul and Stephen W. Kercel. "Sensory substitution and the human-machine interface," *Trends in Cognitive Sciences* 7 (2003): 541–546.

Ballard, Dana, M. Hayhoe, P. K. Pook, and R. P. Rao. "Deictic codes for the embodiment of cognition," *Behavioral and Brain Sciences* 20 (1997): 723–767.

Baricco, Alessandro. *L'anima di Hegel e le mucche del Wisconsin: Una riflessione su musica colta e modernità*, Milan: Garzanti, 1992.

Baron-Cohen, Simon. "The cognitive neuroscience of autism: Evolutionary approaches," in Michael S. Gazzaniga (ed.), *The new cognitive neurosciences*, pp. 1249–1258.

Barthes, Roland. "La mode et les sciences humaines," *Échanges* (August, 1966).

Barthes, Roland. *Système de la mode*, Paris: Le Seuil, 1967.

Bartra, Roger. "La conciencia y el exocerebro," *Letras Libres* (Spanish edition) 29 (2004): 34–39.

Bartra, Roger. "El exocerebro: Una hipótesis sobre la conciencia," *Ludus Vitalis* 23 (2005): 103–115.

Bartra, Roger. *Melancholy and culture: Diseases of the soul in Golden Age Spain*, Iberian and Latin American Studies series, Cardiff: University of Wales Press, 2008.

Bateson, Gregory. *Steps to an ecology of mind*, University of Chicago Press, 1972.

Bateson, Patrick. "Theories of play," in Anthony D. Pellegrini, *The Oxford handbook of the development of play*, Oxford University Press, 2011.

Baynes, Kathleen and Michael S. Gazzaniga. "Consciousness, introspection, and the split-brain: The two minds/one body problem," in Gazzaniga (ed.), *The new cognitive neurosciences*, pp. 1355–1363.

Bentivoglio, Marina. "Cortical structure and mental skills: Oskar Vogt and the legacy of Lenin's brain," *Brain Research Bulletin* 47 (1998): 291–296.

Bergson, Henri. *Le rire: Essai sur la signification du comique*, Paris: F. Alcan, 1924.

Bernstein, Leonard. *The unanswered question*, Cambridge, MA: Harvard University Press, 1976.

Berntson, Gary G. and John T. Cacioppo. "From homeostasis to allodynamic regulation," in *Handbook of psychophysiology*, 2nd edn., Cambridge University Press, 2000.

Bever, T. G. "The nature of cerebral dominance in speech behavior of the child and adult," in R. Huxley and R. Ingham (eds.), *Language acquisition: Models and methods*, London: Academic Press, 1971.

Blackmore, Susan. *Conversations on consciousness*, New York: Oxford University Press, 2006.

Blackmore, Susan. *The meme machine*, Oxford University Press, 1999.

Bor, Daniel. *The ravenous brain: How the new science of consciousness explains our insatiable search for meaning*, New York: Basic Books, 2012.

Brailowsky, Simón. *Las sustancias de los sueños: Neuropsicofarmacología*, Mexico: Fondo de Cultura Económica, 1995.

Brillat-Savarin, Jean Anthelme. *Physiologie du goût, ou, méditations de gastronomie transcendante*, Paris: Just Tessier, Libraire, 1834.

Brown, Donald E. *Human universals*, New York: McGraw-Hill, 1991.

Bruner, Emiliano, Giorgio Manzi, and Juan Luis Asuaga. "Encephalization and allometric trajectories in the genus *Homo*: Evidence from Neanderthal and modern lineages," *Proceedings of the National Academy of Sciences* 100 (26) (2003): 15335–15340.

Budd, Malcolm. *Music and the emotions: The philosophical theories*, London: Routledge, 1985.

Burghardt, Gordon M. "Defining and recognizing play," in Anthony D. Pellegrini, *The Oxford handbook of the development of play*, Oxford University Press, 2011.

Caillois, Roger. *Les jeux et les hommes*, Paris: Gallimard, 1967.

Carmena, José M. *et al.* "Learning to control a brain-machine interface for reaching and grasping by primates," *Public Library of Science-Biology* 1 (2) (October 2003): 1–16.

Caro Baroja, Julio. *Los Baroja*, Madrid: Taurus, 1972.

Cassirer, Ernst. *An essay on man: An introduction to a philosophy of human culture*, New Haven: Yale University Press, 1944.

Cassirer, Ernst. *Myth and language* [1924], translated by Susanne K. Langer, New York: Harper, 1946.

Changeux, Jean-Pierre. *L'homme de vérité*, Paris: Odile Jacob, 2002.

Changeux, Jean-Pierre and Paul Ricoeur. *Ce qui nous fait penser; La nature et la règle*, Paris: Odile Jacob, 1998.

Chapin, Heather, Epifanio Bagarinao, and Sean Mackey. "Real-time fMRI applied to pain management," *Neuroscience Letters* 520, no. 2 (2012): 174–181.

Chomsky, Noam. "Linguistics and politics," *New Left Review* 57 (1969): 21–34.

Chomsky, Noam. *New horizons in the study of language and mind*, New York: Cambridge University Press, 2000.

Churchland, Patricia. *Braintrust: What neuroscience tells us about morality*, Princeton University Press, 2011.

Churchland, Paul. "Rules, know-how, and the future of moral cognition," in *Neurophilosophy at work*, Cambridge University Press, 2007.

Churchland, Paul. "Toward a cognitive neurobiology of moral virtues," in *Neurophilosophy at work*, Cambridge University Press, 2007.

Clark, Andy. *Being there: Putting brain, body, and world together again*, Cambridge, MA: MIT Press, 1997.

Clark, Andy. *Natural-born cyborgs: Minds, technologies, and the future of human intelligence*, Oxford University Press, 2003.

Clark, Andy. *Supersizing the mind: Embodiment, action, and the cognitive extension*, Oxford University Press, 2008.

Clark, Andy. "Word and action: Reconciling rules and know-how in moral cognition," in R. Campbell and B. Hunter (eds.), *Moral epistemology naturalized*, University of Calgary Press, 2000.

Clark, Andy and David Chalmers. "The extended mind," appendix to Andy Clark, *Supersizing the mind: Embodiment, action, and the cognitive extension*, Oxford University Press, 2008.

Clark, Thomas W. "Fear of mechanism: A compatibilist critique of the 'volitional brain'," in Benjamin Libet, Anthony Freeman, and Keith Sutherland (eds.), *The volitional brain: Towards a neuroscience of free will*, Exeter: Imprint Academic, 1999.

Clifford, Erin. "Neural plasticity: Merzenich, Taub, and Greenough," *Harvard Brain* 6 (1999): 16–20.

Cooke, Deryck. *The language of music*, Oxford University Press, 1959.

Crick, Francis. *The astonishing hypothesis*, New York: Scribner, 1993.

Crick, Francis and Christof Koch. "A framework for consciousness," *Nature* 6 (2003): 119–126.

Curtiss, Susan. *Genie: A psycholinguistic story of a modern "wild child,"* New York: Academic Press, 1977.

Damasio, Antonio. *Descartes' error: Emotion, reason, and the human brain*, New York: Putnam, 1994.

Damasio, Antonio. *The feeling of what happens: Body and emotion in the making of consciousness*, New York: Harcourt Brace, 1999.

Damasio, Antonio. *Looking for Spinoza: Joy, sorrow, and the feeling brain*, Orlando: Harcourt, 2003.

Damasio, Antonio. *Self comes to mind: Constructing the conscious brain*, New York: Pantheon Books, 2010.

Dawkins, Richard. *The selfish gene*, 2nd edn., Oxford University Press, 1989.

de la Mare, Heidi. "Domesticity in dispute," in Irene Cieraad (ed.), *At home: An anthropology of domestic space*, Syracuse University Press, 1999.

Deecke, Lüder and Hans Helmut Kornhuber. "Human freedom, reasoned will, and the brain: The Bereitschaftspotential," in Marjan Jahanshahi and Mark Hallett (eds.), *The Bereitschaftspotential: Movement-related cortical potentials* New York: Kluwer Academic/Plenun Publishers, 2003.

Dehaene, Stanislas. "Les bases cérébrales d'une acquisition culturelle: La lecture," in Jean-Pierre Changeux (ed.), *Gènes et culture*, Paris: Odile Jacob, 2003.

Dehaene, Stanislas. *The number sense: How the mind creates mathematics*, revised 2nd edn., Oxford University Press, 1997.

Delaporte, Yves. "Le signe vestimentaire," *L'Homme* 20, no. 3 (1980): 109–142.

Delaporte, Yves. "Le vêtement dans les sociétés traditionelles," in Jean Poirier (ed.), *Histoire des mœurs*, vol. I, Encyclopédie de la Pléiade, Paris: Gallimard, 1990.

Delius, Juan. "The nature of culture," in M. S. Dawkins, T. R. Halliday, and R. Dawkins (eds.), *The Tinbergen legacy*, London: Chapman & Hall, 1991.

Dennett, Daniel C. *Consciousness explained*, Boston: Little, Brown & Co., 1991.

Dennett, Daniel C. *Freedom evolves*, London: Penguin Books, 2004.

Dennett, Daniel C. *Sweet dreams: Philosophical obstacles to a science of consciousness*, Cambridge, MA: MIT Press, 2005.

Diamond, M. C. *et al.* "On the brain of a scientist: Albert Einstein," *Experimental Neurology* 88 (1985): 198–204.

Díaz, José Luis. "El cerebro moral, la voluntad y la neuroética," in Juliana Gonzalez and Jorge Enrique Linares (eds.), *Diálogos de ética y bioética*, Mexico: Fondo de Cultura Económica, 2013.

Díaz, José Luis. "Subjetividad y método: La condición científica de la conciencia y de los informes en primera persona," in C. Torner Aguilar and J. Velázquez Moctezuma (eds.), *Tópicos en la psiquiatría biológica*, Mexico: Universidad Autónoma Metropolitana, 2000.

Dickinson, Emily. *The Complete Poems of Emily Dickinson*, edited by Thomas H. Johnson. Boston: Little, Brown, 1960.

Doidge, Norman. *The brain that changes itself*, London: Penguin Books, 2007.

Donald, Merlin. *A mind so rare: The evolution of human consciousness*, New York: Norton, 2001.

Donald, Merlin. *Origins of the modern mind: Three stages in the evolution of culture and cognition*, Cambridge, MA: Harvard University Press, 1991.

Doupe, Allison J. *et al.* "The song system: Neural circuits essential throughout life for vocal behavior and plasticity," in Gazzaniga (ed.), *The new cognitive neurosciences*, pp. 451–468.

Draaisma, Douwe. *Metaphors of memory: A history of ideas about the mind*, Cambridge University Press, 2000.

Duerr, Hans Peter. *Nudité et pudeur: Le mythe du processus de civilisation*, Paris: Éditions de la Maison des Sciences de l'Homme, 1990.

Eagleman, David. *Incognito: The secret lives of the brain*, Edinburgh: Canongate, 2011.

Eccles, John C. *How the self controls its brain*, Berlin: Springer-Verlag, 1994.

Edelman, Gerald M. *Bright air, brilliant fire: On the matter of the mind*, New York: Basic Books, 1992.

Edelman, Gerald M. *Wider than the sky: The phenomenal gift of consciousness*, New Haven: Yale University Press, 2004.

Edelman, Gerald and Giulio Tononi. *A universe of consciousness: How matter becomes imagination*, New York: Basic Books, 2000.

Eibl-Eibesfeld, Irenäus. *Human ethology*, New York: Aldine de Gruyter, 1989.

Einon, Dorothy and Michael Potegal. "Enhanced defense in adult rats deprived of playfighting experience as juveniles," *Aggressive Behavior* 17 (1): 27–40, 1991.

Eiseley, Loren. *Darwin's century: Evolution and the men who discovered it*, New York: Doubleday Anchor Books, 1961.

Erikson, Erik H. "Play and actuality," in Maria W. Piers (ed.), *Play and development*, New York: Norton, 1972.

Fadiga, Luciano, *et al.* "Motor facilitation during action observation: A magnetic stimulation study," *Journal of Neurophysiology* 73 (1995): 2608–2611.

Fagen, Robert. *Animal play behaviour*, Oxford University Press, 1981.

Faubion, James D. *An anthropology of ethics*, New York: Cambridge University Press, 2011.

Fernald, Russell D. and Stephanie A. White. "Social control of brains: From behavior to genes," in Gazzaniga (ed.), *The new cognitive neurosciences*, pp. 1193–1209.

Fields, R. Douglas. "Making memories stick," *Scientific American* 292 (2005): 74–81.

Fields, R. Douglas. "The other half of the brain," *Scientific American* 290 (2004): 26–33.

Fischer, Roland. "Why the mind is not in the head but in society's connectionist network," *Diogenes* 151 (1990): 1–27.

Fodor, Jerry. *The modularity of mind*, Cambridge, MA: MIT Press, 1983.

Fodor, Jerry. "Where is my mind?" *London Review of Books* (February 12, 2009).

Fogassi, Leonardo and Vittorio Gallese. "The neural correlates of action understanding in non-human primates," in Maxim I. Stamenov and Vittorio Gallese (eds.), *Mirror neurons and the evolution of brain and language*, Amsterdam: John Benjamins, 2002.

Fourastié, Jean. *Le rire, suite*, Paris: Denoël-Gonthier, 1983.

Fox, Christopher. *Locke and the Scriblerians: Identity and consciousness in early eighteenth century Britain*, Berkeley: University of California Press, 1988.

Galanter, Eugene and Murray Gerstenhaber. "On thought: The extrinsic theory," *Psychological Review* 63 (4) (1956): 218–227.

Gallagher, Shaun. "Where's the action? Epiphenomenalism and the problem of free will," in W. Banks, S. Pockett, and S. Gallagher (eds.), *Does consciousness cause behavior? An investigation of the nature of volition*, Cambridge, MA: MIT Press, 2006.

Gazzaniga, Michael S. *The ethical brain*, New York: Dana Press, 2005.

Gazzaniga, Michael S. *The mind's past*, Berkeley: University of California Press, 1998.

Gazzaniga, Michael S. *The social brain: Discovering the networks of the mind*, New York: Basic Books, 1985.

Gazzaniga, Michael S. (ed.). *The new cognitive neurosciences*, 2nd edn., Cambridge, MA: MIT Press, 2000.

Geertz, Clifford. "Culture, mind, brain / Brain, mind, culture," in *Available light: Anthropological reflections on philosophical topics*, Princeton University Press, 2000.

Geertz, Clifford. *The interpretation of cultures*, New York: Basic Books, 1973.

Gellner, Ernest. *Language and solitude: Wittgenstein, Malinowski and the Habsburg dilemma*, Cambridge University Press, 1998.

Gershon, Michael D. *The second brain*, New York: HarperCollins, 1998.

Glanville, B. B., C. T. Best, and R. Levenson. "A cardiac measure of cerebral asymmetries in infant auditory perception," *Developmental Psychology* 13 (1977): 54–59.

Goldberg, Elkhonon. *The executive brain: Frontal lobes and the civilized mind*, Oxford University Press, 2001.

Gönzü, Artin and Suzanne Gaskins. "Comparing and extending Piaget's and Vygotsky's understandings of play: Symbolic as individual, sociocultural, and educational interpretation," in Anthony D. Pellegrini (ed.), *The Oxford handbook of the development of play*, Oxford University Press, 2011.

Goody, Jack. *The development of the family and marriage in Europe*, Cambridge University Press, 1983.

Gould, Stephen Jay. *Ontogeny and phylogeny*, Cambridge, MA: Harvard University Press, 1977.

Gould, Stephen Jay. *The structure of evolutionary theory*, Cambridge, MA: Harvard University Press, 2000.

Gould, Stephen Jay and S. Vrba. "Exaptation: A missing term in the science of form," *Paleobiology* 8 (1982): 4–15.

Graham Brown, Thomas. "The intrinsic factors in the act of progression in the mammal," *Proceedings of the Royal Society, B Biological Sciences*, 84 (1911): 308–319.

Gray, Jeffrey. "It's time to move from philosophy to science," *Journal of Consciousness Studies* 9 (11) (2002): 49–52.

Griffiths, Timothy D. "Musical hallucinosis in acquired deafness: Phenomenology and brain substrate," *Brain* 123 (2000): 2065–2076.

Groos, Karl. *Die Spiele der Menschen*, Jena: Verlag von Gustav Fischer, 1899.

Groos, Karl. *Die Spiele der Thiere*, Jena: Verlag von Gustav Fischer, 1896.

Habermas, Jürgen. "Symbolic expression and ritual behavior: Ernst Cassirer and Arnold Gehlen revisited," *Time of transitions*, Cambridge: Polity, 2006.

Haidt, Jonathan. *The righteous mind: Why good people are divided by politics and religion*, New York: Pantheon, 2012.

Hallett, Mark. "Volitional control of movement: The psychology of free will," *Clinical Neurophysiology* 118 (2007): 1179–1192.

Harnad, Stevan. "Correlation vs. causality: How/why the mind-body problem is hard," *Journal of Consciousness Studies* 7 (4) (2000): 54–61.

Harnad, Stevan. "No easy way out," *The Sciences* 41 (2) (2001): 36–42.

Hauser, Marc D. *Moral minds: How nature designed our universal sense of right and wrong*, New York: HarperCollins, 2006.

Hayek, Friedrich A. *The constitution of liberty* [1960], University of Chicago Press, 2011.

Hayek, Friedrich A. *The sensory order*, London: Routledge & Kegan Paul, 1952.

Hebb, Donald D. *The organization of behavior: A neuropsychological theory*, New York: John Wiley, 1949.

Heidegger, Martin. *The fundamental concepts of metaphysics: World, finitude, solitude*, translated by William McNeill and Nicholas Walker, Bloomington: Indiana University Press, 1995.

Henshilwood, Christopher S. *et al.* "Emergence of modern human behavior: Middle Stone Age engravings in South Africa," *Science* 295 (2002): 1278–1280.

Heusden, Barend von. "Jakob von Uexküll and Ernst Cassirer," *Semiotica* 134 (2001): 275–292.

Hickok, Gregory. "Eight problems for the mirror neuron theory of action understanding in monkeys and humans," *Journal of Cognitive Neuroscience* 21 (2008): 1229–1243.

Hirschfeld, Lawrence A. and Susan A. Gelman (eds.). *Mapping the mind: Domain specificity in cognition and culture*, Cambridge University Press, 1994.

Hofstadter, Douglas. *Gödel, Escher, Bach: An eternal golden braid*, New York: Basic Books, 1999.

Hofstadter, Douglas. *I am a strange loop*, New York: Basic Books, 2007.

Hood, Bruce. *The self illusion: How the social brain creates identity*, Oxford University Press, 2012.

Hubel, D. H. and T. N. Wiesel. "The period of susceptibility to the physiological effects of unilateral eye closure in kittens," *Journal of Physiology* 206 (1970): 419–436.

Huizinga, Johan. *Homo ludens*, translation by Eugenio Imaz, Madrid: Alianza Editorial, 1972.

Hume, David. *An enquiry concerning human understanding*, New York: Oxford University Press, 2007.

Hume, David. *A treatise of human nature*, Oxford University Press, 1978.

Humphrey, Nicholas. "How to solve the mind-body problem," *Journal of Consciousness Studies* 7 (4) (2000): 5–20.

Iacoboni, Marco. *Mirroring people: The science of empathy and how we connect with others*, New York: Picador, 2009.

Jackendoff, Ray. *Language, consciousness, culture: Essays on mental structure*, Cambridge, MA: MIT Press, 2007.

Jackson, Franck. "Epiphenomenal qualia," *Philosophical Quarterly* 32 (1982): 127–136.

Jaeger, Werner. *Paideia: The ideals of Greek culture*, Vol. III: *The conflict of cultural ideals in the age of Plato*, trans. Gilbert Highet. Oxford University Press, 1986.

Jakobson, Roman. "Two aspects of language and two types of aphasic disturbances," in R. Jakobson and Morris Halle, *Fundamentals of language*, La Haya: Mouton, 1956.

James, Henry. *The portrait of a lady*, London: Macmillan, 1881.

James, William. *The principles of psychology*, New York: Holt, 1890.

Jaynes, Julian. *The origin of consciousness in the breakdown of the bicameral mind*, Boston: Houghton Mifflin, 1976.

Jones, Peter E. "Contradictions and unanswered questions in the Genie case: a fresh look at the linguistic evidence," *Language & Communication* 15 (3) (1995): 261–280.

Jones, William Jervis. *German Kinship Terms, (750–1500)*, Berlin: de Gruyer, 1980.

Jouary, Jean-Paul. *Ferran Adrià, l'art des mets: Un philosophe à el Bulli*, Paris: Les Impressions Nouvelles, 2011.

Kanner, Leo. "Autistic disturbances of affective contact," *Nervous Child* 2 (1943): 217–250.

Katz, Lawrence C. *et al.* "Activity and the development of the visual cortex: New perspectives," in Gazzaniga (ed.), *The new cognitive neurosciences*, pp. 199–212.

Keller, Helen. *The story of my life* [1903], restored edition that includes several letters, texts by Anne Sullivan, John Albert Macy and two essays by Roger Shattuck as supplements, New York: Norton, 2003.

Keller, Helen. *The world I live in* [1908], New York: New York Review of Books, 2003.

Kennepohl, Stephan. "Toward a cultural neuropsychology: An alternative view and preliminary model," *Brain and Cognition* 41 (1999): 366–380.

Kimura, Doreen. "Speech lateralization in young children as determined by an auditory test," *Journal of Comparative and Physiological Psychology* 56 (1963): 899–902.

Koch, Christof. *Consciousness: Confessions of a romantic reductionist*, Cambridge, MA: MIT Press, 2012.

Koch, Christof. *The quest for consciousness: A neurobiological approach*, Englewood, CO: Roberts & Company, 2004.

Koch, Christof and Francis Crick. "Some thoughts on consciousness and neuroscience," in Gazzaniga (ed.), *The new cognitive neurosciences*.

Korsmeyer, Carolyn. *Making sense of taste: Food and philosophy*, Ithaca: Cornell University Press, 1999.

Kuhl, Patricia K. "Language, mind, and brain: Experience alters perception," in Gazzaniga (ed.), *The new cognitive neurosciences*, pp. 99–115.

Kuper, Adam. *The chosen primate: Human nature and cultural diversity*, Cambridge, MA: Harvard University Press, 1994.

Kuper, Adam. "If memes are the answer, what is the question?" in Robert Aunger (ed.), *Darwinizing culture: The status of memetics as a science*, Oxford University Press, 2000.

Langer, Susanne K. *Philosophy in a new key: A study in the symbolism of reason, rite, and art* [1942], Cambridge, MA: Harvard University Press, 1957.

Leiber, Justin. "Nature's experiments, society's closures," *Journal of the Theory of Social Behavior* 27 (2002): 325–343.

Lévi-Strauss, Claude. *Le totémisme aujourd'hui*, Paris: Presses Universitaires de France, 1962.

Lewontin, Richard. *Biology as ideology*, New York: HarperCollins, 1993.

Li, Charles N. and Jean-Marie Hombert. "On the evolutionary origin of language," in Maxim I. Stamenov and Vittorio Gallese (eds.), *Mirror neurons and the evolution of brain and language*, Amsterdam: John Benjamins, 2002.

Libet, Benjamin. "Do we have free will?" in Benjamin Libet, Anthony Freeman and Keith Sutherland (eds.), *The volitional brain: Towards a neuroscience of free will*, Exeter: Imprint Academic, 1999.

Llinás, Rodolfo R. *I of the vortex: From neurons to self*, Cambridge, MA: MIT Press, 2002.

Locke, John. *An essay concerning human understanding*, 2nd edn., London: Thomas Dring, 1694.

Lorenzo, Guillermo. "El origen del lenguaje como sobresalto natural," *Ludus Vitalis* 17 (2002): 175–193.

Luria, Alexandr Romanovich. *Language and cognition*, New York: Wiley, 1981.

Luria, Alexandr Romanovich. *The man with a shattered world: The history of a brain wound*, Cambridge, MA: Harvard University Press, 2004.

Luria, Alexandr Romanovich. *The mind of a mnemonist*, New York: Basic Books, 1968.

Luria, Alexandr Romanovich. *The neuropsychology of memory*, New York: Winston, 1976.

MacLean, Paul D. *A triune concept of brain and behaviour*, University of Toronto Press, 1969.

Martin, Emily. "Mind-body problems," *American Ethnologist* 27 (3) (2000): 569–590.

Martin, Kelsey C., Dusan Bartsch, Craig H. Bailey, and Eric R. Kandel. "Molecular mechanisms underlying learning-related long lasting synaptic plasticity," in Gazzaniga (ed.), *The new cognitive neurosciences*, pp. 121–137.

McEwen, Bruce S. "Stress, sex, and the structural and functional plasticity of the hippocampus," in Gazzaniga (ed.), *The new cognitive neurosciences*, pp. 171–197.

McGinn, Colin. *The mysterious flame: Conscious minds in a material world*, New York: Basic Books, 1999.

McLuhan, Marshall. "A candid conversation with the high priest of popcult and metaphysician of media," interview in *Playboy*, March 1969, reproduced in Eric McLuhan and Frank Zingrone (eds.), *Essential McLuhan*, New York: Basic Books, 1995.

McLuhan, Marshall. *Understanding media: The extensions of man*, New York: McGraw-Hill, 1964.

Mele, Alfred R. "Decision, intentions, urges, and free will: Why Libet has not shown what he says he has," in Joseph Keim Campbell, Michael O'Rourke and Harry Silverstein (eds.), *Causation and explanation*, Boston: MIT Press, 2007.

Merleau-Ponty, Maurice. *Nature: Course notes from the Collège de France*, Evanston: Northwestern University Press, 2003.

Merleau-Ponty, Maurice. *Phénoménologie de la perception*, Paris: Gallimard, 1945.

Mithen, Steve. *The prehistory of the mind: The cognitive origins of art, religion and science*, London: Thames and Hudson, 1996.

Mithen, Steve. *The singing Neanderthals: The origins of music, language, mind and body*, Cambridge, MA: Harvard University Press, 2006.

Moreno-Armella, Luis and Stephen J. Hegedus. "Co-action with digital technologies," *ZDM Mathematics Education* 41 (2009): 505–519.

Morrot, Gill, Fréderic Brochet, and Denis Duboudieu. "The color of odors," *Brain and Language* 79 (2001): 309–320.

Mountcastle, Vernon B. "Brain science at the century's ebb," *Dædalus* 127 (2) (1998): 1–36.

Neville, Helen J. and Daphne Bavelier. "Specificity and plasticity in neurocognitive development in humans," in Gazzaniga (ed.), *The new cognitive neurosciences*, pp. 83–98.

North, Douglass. *Understanding the process of economic change*, Princeton University Press, 2005.

O'Regan, J. Kevin. "Solving the 'real' mysteries of visual perception: The world as an outside memory," *Canadian Journal of Psychology* 46: 461–488, 1992.

Orr, H. Allen. "Darwinian storytelling," *New York Review of Books* (February 27, 2003).

Ortega y Gasset, José. *Meditaciones del Quijote*, edited by Julián Marías, Madrid: Cátedra, 1990.

Paterniti, Michael. *Driving Mr. Albert: A trip across America with Einstein's brain*, New York: Dial Press, 2000.

Pellis, Sergio M. and Vivien C. Pellis. "Rough-and-tumble play and the development of the social brain," *Current Directions in Psychological Science* 16 (2) (2007): 95–98.

Piaget, Jean. *La formation du symbole chez l'enfant: Imitation, jeu et rêve. Image et représentation*, Neuchâtel: Delchaux & Niestlé, 1945.

Piattelli-Palmarini, Massimo (ed.). *Théories du langage, théories de l'apprentissage: Le débat entre Jean Piaget et Noam Chomsky*, Paris: Seuil, 1979.

Pinker, Steven. *The blank slate*, New York: Penguin, 2002.

Pinker, Steven and H. Allen Orr. "The blank slate: An exchange," *New York Review of Books* (May 1, 2003).

Pons, Tim, P. E. Garraghty, A. K. Ommaya, J. H. Kaas, E. Taub, and M. Mishkin. "Massive cortical reorganization after sensory deafferentation in adult macaques," *Science* 252 (1991): 1857–1860.

Popper, Karl R. and John C. Eccles. *The self and its brain*, Berlin: Springer-Verlag, 1977.

Popper, Karl, B. I. B. Lindahl, and P. Århem. "A discussion of the mind-brain problem," *Theoretical Medicine* 14 (1993): 167–180.

Pratt, Carroll C. *The meaning of music*, New York: McGraw-Hill, 1931.

Prigogine, Ilya. "The rediscovery of value and the opening of economics," in Kurt Dopfer (ed.), *The evolutionary foundations of economics*, Cambridge University Press, 2005.

Putnam, Hilary. *The threefold cord: Mind, body, and world*, New York: Columbia University Press, 1999.

Raine, Adrian, Todd Lencz, Susan Bihrle, Lori LaCasse, and Patrick Colletti. "Reduced prefrontal gray matter volume and reduced autonomic activity in antisocial personality disorder," in John T. Cacioppo *et al.* (eds.), *Foundations of social neuroscience*, Cambridge, MA: MIT Press, 2002.

Ramachandran, Vilayanur S. *A brief tour of human consciousness*, New York: Pi Press, 2004.

Ramachandran, Vilayanur S. *The tell-tale brain: A neuroscientist's quest for what makes us human*, New York: Norton, 2011.

Ramachandran, Vilayanur S., and Sandra Blakeslee. *Phantoms in the brain: Human nature and the architecture of the mind*, London: Fourth Estate, 1998.

Ramachandran, Vilayanur S., and Edward M. Hubbard. "Hearing colors, tasting shapes," *Scientific American* 288 (2003): 43–49.

Ramón y Cajal, Santiago. "La rétine des vertébrés," *La Cellule* 9 (1893): 119–257.

Rapoport, Judith. *The boy who couldn't stop washing: The experience and treatment of obsessive-compulsive disorder*, London: Fontana, 1990.

Rawls, John. *A theory of justice*, Cambridge, MA: Harvard University Press, 1971.

Reyna, Stephen P. *Connections: Brain, mind, and culture in a social anthropology*, London: Routledge, 2002.

Rheims, Maurice. "Histoire du mobilier," in Jean Poirier (ed.), *Histoire des mœurs*, vol. I, Encyclopédie de la Pléiade, Paris: Gallimard, 1990.

Ribeiro, Aileen. *Dress and morality*, London: B. T. Batsford, 1986.

Rimbaud, Arthur. *Œuvres complètes*, Bibliothèque de la Pléiade, Paris: Gallimard, 1972.

Rizzolatti, Giacomo and Michael A. Arbib. "Language within our grasp," *Trends in Neurosciences* 21 (1998): 188–194.

Rizzolatti, Giacomo, L. Fadiga, L. Fogassi, and V. Gallese. "Premotor cortex and the recognition of the motor actions," *Cognitive Brain Research* 3 (1996): 131–141.

Romo, Ranulfo, Adrián Hernández, and Emilio Salinas. "Neurobiología de la toma de decisiones," in Ramón de la Fuente (ed.), *Aportaciones recientes de la biología a la psiquiatría*, Mexico: El Colegio Nacional, 2003.

Rose, Steven. *Lifelines: Biology beyond determinism*, New York: Oxford University Press, 1998.

Rosen, Charles. *Arnold Schoenberg*, New York: Viking Press, 1975.

Rosenblueth, Arturo. *Mind and brain: A philosophy of science*, Cambridge, MA: MIT Press, 1970.

Rousseau, Jean-Jacques. *Discours sur l'origine et les fondemens de l'inegalité parmi les hommes* [1755], Œuvres complètes, vol. III, Paris: Gallimard, 1964.

Rymer, Russ. *Genie: An abused child's flight from silence*, New York: HarperCollins, 1993.

Sacks, Oliver. "An anthropologist on Mars," in *An anthropologist on Mars: Seven paradoxical tales*, New York: Knopf, 1995.

Sacks, Olivier. *Awakenings*, New York: Vintage, 1999.
Savage-Rumbaugh, Sue and Roger Lewin. *Kanzi: The ape at the brink of the human mind*, New York: Wiley, 1994.
Schiller, Friedrich. *Letters upon the aesthetic education of man* [1794], Raleigh, NC: Hayes Barton Press, 1990.
Schwartz, Jeffrey M. "A role for volition and attention in the generation of new brain circuitry: Towards a neurobiology of mental force," in Benjamin Libet, Anthony Freeman and Keith Sutherland (eds.), *The volitional brain: Towards a neuroscience of free will*, Exeter: Imprint Academic, 1999.
Searle, John R. *The construction of social reality*, New York: Penguin Books, 1995.
Searle, John R. *Freedom and neurobiology: Reflections on free will, language, and political power*, New York: Columbia University Press, 2004.
Searle, John R. *Mind: A brief introduction*, Oxford University Press, 2004.
Selye, Hans. "Homeostasis and heterostasis," *Perspectives in Biology and Medicine* 16 (1973): 441–445.
Schatz, C. J. "The developing brain," *Scientific American* 267 (1992): 60–67.
Sheldrake, Rupert. *The presence of the past: Morphic resonance and the habits of nature*, New York: Vintage, 1989.
Shepherd, Gordon M. *Neurogastronomy: How the brain creates flavor and why it matters*, New York: Columbia University Press, 2012.
Skinner, Burrhus F. *About behaviorism*, New York: Knopf, 1974.
Smith, Adam. *The theory of moral sentiments*. London: Henry G. Bohn, 1853.
Smith, Marcia Datlow and Ronald G. Belcher. "Facilitated communication: The effects of facilitator knowledge and level of assistance on output," *Journal of Autism and Developmental Disorders*, 24 (3) (1994): 357–367.
Spang, Michael *et al.* "Your own hall of memories," *Scientific American Mind* 16 (2) (2005): 60–65.
Sperber, Dan. "Contre certains a priori anthropologiques," in Edgar Morin and M. Piatelli-Palmarini (eds.), *L'unité de l'homme: Invariants biologiques et universaux culturels*, Paris: Le Seuil, 1974.
Sperber, Dan. "The modularity of thought and the epidemiology of representations," in Lawrence A. Hirschfeld and Susan A. Gelman (eds.), *Mapping the mind: Domain specificity in cognition and culture*, Cambridge University Press, 1994.
Sperry, Roger W. "Hemisphere deconnection and unity in conscious awareness," *American Psychologist* 23 (1968): 723–733.
Spinoza, Baruch. *Ethics, demonstrated in geometrical order*, translated by R. H. M. Elwes, Project Gutenberg e-book.
Squicciarino, Nicola. *Il vestito parla: Considerazioni psicosociologiche sull'abbigliamento*, Rome: Armando, 1986.
Squire, Larry R. and Barbara J. Knowlton. "The medial temporal lobe, the hippocampus, and the memory systems of the brain," in Gazzaniga (ed.), *The new cognitive neurosciences*, pp. 765–779.
Stamenov, Maxim I. "Some features that make mirror neurons and human language faculty unique," in Maxim I. Stamenov and Vittorio Gallese (eds.), *Mirror neurons and the evolution of brain and language*, Amsterdam: John Benjamins, 2002.
Storr, Anthony. *Music and the mind*, London: Collins, 1992.
Tagore, Rabindranath. "Three conversations: Tagore talks with Einstein, with Rolland, and Wells," *Asia*, 31 (3) (March, 1931): 138–143.

Tattersall, Ian. *The monkey in the mirror: Essays on the science of what makes us human*, San Diego: Harcourt, 2002.

Taylor, Lou. *The study of dress history*, Manchester University Press, 2002.

Thaut, Michael H. *Rhythm, music, and the brain: Scientific foundations and clinical applications*, New York: Routledge, 2005.

Tomasello, Michael. *The cultural origins of human cognition*, Cambridge, MA: Harvard University Press, 1999.

Tononi, Giulio. "Consciousness as integrated information: A provisional manifesto," *The Biological Bulletin* 215 (December, 2008): 216–243.

Tooby, John and Leda Cosmides. "The psychological foundations of culture," in J. H. Barkow, L. Cosmides and J. Tooby, *The adapted mind*, New York: Oxford University Press, 1992.

Tort, Patrick. *La raison classificatoire*, Paris: Aubier, 1989.

Tranel, Daniel, Antoine Bechara, and Antonio R. Damasio. "Decision making and the somatic marker hypothesis," in Gazzaniga (ed.), *The new cognitive neurosciences*, pp. 1047–1061.

Treffert, Darold A. *Extraordinary people: Understanding savant syndrome*, Lincoln, NE: iUniverse.com, 2000.

Treffert, Darold A. and Gregory L. Wallace. "Island of genius," *Scientific American* (June 2002).

Uexküll, Jakob von. *Ideas para una concepción biológica del mundo* [*Bausteine zu einer biologischen Weltanschauung. Gesemelte Aufsätze*, 1913], Madrid: Calpe, 1922.

Uexküll, Jakob von. *Meditaciones biológicas: La teoría de la significación* [Bedeutungslehr, 1940], Madrid: Revista de Occidente, 1942.

Uexküll, Jakob von. "A stroll through the worlds of animals and men," in *German essays on science in the 20th century* (The German Library 82), New York: Continuum, 1996.

Utekhin, Ilia. "Spanish echoes of Jakob von Uexküll's thought," *Semiotica* 134 (2001): 635–642.

Varela, Francisco J. "The reenchantment of the concrete," in J. Crary and S. Kwinter (eds.), *Incorporations*, New York: Zone Books, 1992.

Varela, Francisco J., Evan T. Thompson, and Eleanor Rosch. *The embodied mind*, Cambridge, MA: MIT Press, 1991.

Velmans, Max. "How could conscious experiences affect brains?" *Journal of Consciousness Studies* 9 (11) (2002): 3–29.

Vuilleumier, P. *et al.* "Neural fate on seen and unseen faces in visuospatial neglect: A combined event-related MRI and event-related potential study," *Proceedings of the National Academy of Science* (USA) 98 (2001): 3495–3500.

Vygotsky, Lev. "Play and its role in the mental development of the child," *Soviet Psychology* 5 (3) (1967): 6–18.

Vygotsky, Lev. *Thought and language*, revised version by Alex Kozulin, Cambridge, MA: MIT Press, 1986.

Wallace, Alfred Russell. "Darwinism applied to men," in *Darwinism*, London: 1889.

Walter, Henric. *Neurophilosophy of free will: From libertarian illusions to a concept of natural autonomy*, Cambridge, MA: MIT Press, 2001.

Wandell, Brian A. "Computational neuroimaging: Color representations and processing," in Gazzaniga (ed.), *The new cognitive neurosciences*, pp. 291–303.

Weber, Andreas. "Mimesis and metaphor: The biosemiotic generation of meaning in Cassirer and Uexküll," *Sign Systems Studies* 32 (2004): 297–307.

Wegner, Daniel M. *The illusion of conscious will*, Cambridge, MA: MIT Press, 2002.

Welters, Linda (ed.). *Folk dress in Europe and Anatolia: Beliefs about protection and fertility*, Oxford: Berg, 1999.

Wiener, Norbert. *Cybernetics*, 2nd edn, Cambridge, MA: MIT Press, 1961.

Wilson, Robert A. *Boundaries of the mind: The individual in the fragile sciences*, Cambridge University Press, 2004.

Wittgenstein, Ludwig. *Philosophical Investigations / Philosophische Untersuchungen*, Oxford: Blackwell, 1953.

Wittgenstein, Ludwig. *Zettel*, edited by G. E. M. Anscombe and G. H. von Wright, Mexico: Universidad Nacional Autónoma de México, 1979.

Wong, Kate. "The morning of the modern mind," *Scientific American* 292 (6) (2005): 64–73.

Yates, Frances A. *The art of memory*, London: Routledge & Kegan Paul, 1966.

Zahan, Dominique. "L'homme et la couleur," in Jean Poirier (ed.), *Histoire des mœurs*, vol. I, Paris: Encyclopédie de la Pléiade, 1990.

Zatorre, Robert J. and Pascal Belin. "Spectral and temporal processing in human auditory cortex," *Cerebral Cortex* 11 (2001): 946–953.

Index